Living Canvas

Your Total Guide to
TATTOOS, PIERCINGS,
and BODY MODIFICATION

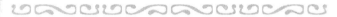

Karen L. Hudson

Living Canvas
Your Total Guide to Tattoos, Piercings, and Body Modification

Published by
Seal Press
A Member of the Perseus Books Group
1700 Fourth Street
Berkeley, California

Library of Congress Cataloging-in-Publication Data

Hudson, Karen L.
  Living canvas : your total guide to tattoos, piercing, and body modification / Karen L. Hudson.
     p. cm.
  Includes bibliographical references.
  ISBN 978-1-58005-288-7
  1. Tattooing. 2. Body piercing. 3. Body painting. I. Title.
  GT2345.H85 2009
  391.6'5—dc22
                    2009004842

Cover and Interior design by Domini Dragoone
Printed in the United States of America by Maple-Vail
Distributed by Publishers Group West

To the children who have suffered because no one was there to teach them what they needed to know.

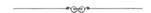

In memory of Daniel Hindle Anderson.

contents

∾ Part two: Body Piercings

✦ Part three: Other Body Modifications and Temporary Art

what is a tattoo?

I'll bet when you hear the word "tattoo," the first thing that comes to mind is a picture on someone's skin. That's what this section is about: tattoos as art. But if you look the word up in the dictionary, the definition is a little different. Tattoos were originally military signals, played on drums or trumpets, to alert soldiers or sailors to return to their barracks. So how did we come to the current understanding of the word "tattoo"—meaning a mark or picture in skin?

There are several theories. One is that the word comes from the Polynesian word *tatoa,* which means "to tap." This certainly makes sense, seeing as the first tattoos were done with sticks and a group of needles that would repeatedly tap color into the skin.

Another common idea is that the word originated from the Tahitian language. When the famed British explorer Captain Cook inquired about the designs he saw on the Tahitian natives, their answer was "*tatau.*" Even this theory has variations, though. Most surmise that *tatau* referred to a rhythmic tapping sound. Other sources say that it simply means "to mark." However, one study offered a different view: In Tahitian, the first "ta" represents something done with the hand. Saying this twice, "ta-ta," implies repeating a certain action. And the last sound, "u," means color. Put it all together, and it means a repetitive act with the hand that colors. Yet another source says that none of this is relevant because the word "tattoo" existed long before Captain Cook started using it.

So, history's not always cut-and-dry. Especially when you're talking about something that's been around for centuries as an integral part of almost every ancient culture that's existed on the planet.

At some point, those cultures converged on the practice of body art, and we have what we know as the modern tattoo—something that has changed dramatically in a very short period of time, and in more ways than one.

> *TIP:* Tebori *is the name for traditional Japanese hand tattooing that is still practiced by some artists today. The tool used is very simple—one or two rows of needles attached to a long, straight stick. The artist taps the needles against the skin in a rhythmic motion, implanting the ink into the tissue. Tattooing this way is much more difficult and slower going than with a machine, but is highly respected for its rich history. Many tattoo enthusiasts will seek out a* tebori *master just to experience this ancient art form firsthand.*

CHAPTER 2

120 years
of tattoo evolution

If you want a detailed history of body art in ancient times, there are some great books and websites listed in the Resources section at the back of the book. What I find most interesting about tattoo history, however, are the more recent developments—those that have happened over the past 120 years or so.

It began with the invention of the tattoo machine. In 1876, Thomas Edison patented the "autographic printer," which was intended to be an engraver, not a tattoo machine. But Samuel O'Reilly, an American tattoo artist and cousin to British tattoo artist Tom Riley, was inspired by the engraver design to invent and patent the very first electric tattoo machine, on December 8, 1891. In 1904, Charlie Wagner (Samuel's apprentice and the first American artist to successfully apply cosmetic tattoos) improved on O'Reilly's design and created the dual-coil tattoo machine that has remained virtually unchanged to this day.

With the advent of the electric tattoo machine, tattoo art took an upward swing that's been gaining momentum ever since. In 1905, a quirky man by the name of August "Cap" Coleman entered the scene with his floating tattoo shop—a handmade raft that he used to travel the Ohio

River in search of work. Over the next fifty years, Cap Coleman made a huge impact on the tattoo industry. His bold, graphic flash-art style quickly became a favorite among collectors and artists alike, starting a trend in tattoo art that became known as "Coleman style." He seemed to have insight that a lot of his fellow artists lacked—an understanding of how a certain design should flow with the body and how to create vivid images with very few lines, and less stress and trauma to the skin. He also was one of the first to understand the inner workings of tattoo machines, and was known to tweak and shim them until they were running as smoothly as possible.

Ironically, though, Cap Coleman—as meticulous about his art and his equipment as he was—had an aversion to personal hygiene, sometimes not bathing or washing his clothes for weeks at a time. Apparently, this didn't hurt his business; while the artistic aspect of tattooing was evolving, there was still little thought given to cleanliness and sterilization. It was common for needles and ink to be reused from customer to customer, and the idea of wearing gloves hadn't even been thought of yet.

Despite this, the demand for ink grew, especially among servicemen. Samuel O'Reilly was once quoted as saying, "A sailor without a tattoo is like a ship without grog: not seaworthy." Maritime tattoos were certainly the bread and butter of most artists, and wartime seemed to perpetuate the need for declarative ink. And wartime was aplenty during the twentieth century, as soldiers from World Wars I and II and the Korean and Vietnam wars kept tattoo artists busy. During these periods of conflict and instability, tattoos also became the glue that bonded servicemen, friends, and families for life.

As tattoos' popularity increased, so did the range of clientele. Even upscale aristocrats desired ink as a way to secretly experience the tawdry side of life. In 1936, *Life* magazine declared that 6 percent of Americans were tattooed. On March 4, 1944, Norman Rockwell's famous painting *The Tattooist* appeared on the front cover of *The Saturday Evening Post*. New York's Coney Island had become the nation's hub of tattooing, with little shops popping up everywhere. It seemed that tattoos had reached a virtual climax of success and acceptance—until it all came crashing down.

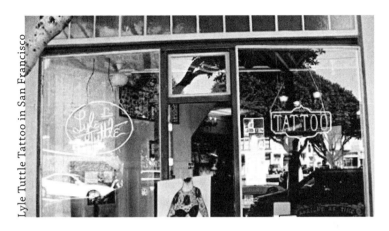

In 1950, the City Council of Norfolk, Virginia, home to the world's largest naval base, declared tattooing "unsanitary and vulgar" and banned the practice, forcing the shutdown of over a dozen shops. In 1961, the city of New York banned tattooing after a breakout of hepatitis B. Once the danger of unsanitary practices was exposed, it almost caused the downfall of the entire industry.

Fortunately, some very important and influential people had entered the tattoo scene just in time to save it from utter destruction. In 1960, Lyle Tuttle opened his shop in San Francisco. Tuttle's talent, experience, self-proclaimed "bullshit artistry," and keen ability to handle the media brought him to the forefront of the trade and caught the attention of many inside and outside the tattoo community.

On October 1, 1970, a most unprecedented event took place: Lyle Tuttle, in all his tattooed glory, appeared on the inside cover of *Rolling Stone* magazine. The three-quarter-page photo preceded a stirring two-page article by Amie Hill entitled "Tattoo Renaissance," in which Hill used her interview with Tuttle as a springboard to create a very positive image of tattooing in a time when the art form was widely considered little less than the work of the Devil himself. That exposure boosted not only Tuttle's celebrity, but also the reputation of the industry as a whole.

Around this time, another influential artist was also making his mark. In 1974, Don Ed Hardy opened the country's first-ever appointment-only custom tattoo shop in San Francisco.

In 1976, the National Tattoo Association (NTA) was formed to heighten "social awareness of tattooing as a contemporary art form." In 1979, the NTA held its first tattoo convention, in Denver, Colorado. Tattoo artists who had once viewed one another as unnecessary competition, and who had guarded their secrets so carefully, were now coming together to share ideas, pushing their profession to new heights and contributing to the creation of a new era of tattoo art.

In 1982, Don Ed Hardy published a series of magazines entitled *TattooTime,* which was hailed as the "tattooer's bible." The very first edition of the magazine, "New Tribalism," showcased the bold, black designs of Bornean and Polynesian tribal tattoo art, which was the catalyst that spurred the demand for the neo-tribal designs that are still so popular today.

By this time, tattooing was turning into a pretty successful moneymaker, and more people wanted in. But the secrets of the masters were still carefully guarded, and it took a lot to squeeze anything valuable out of them without enslaving oneself to them first.

In 1988, Huck Spaulding made both friends and enemies with the publication of his book, *Tattooing A to Z: A Guide to Successful Tattooing.* Spaulding wanted to share his knowledge with the world—and then make a profit selling his tattoo supplies to anyone wanting to give it a try. Now any young hopeful with a shred of artistic talent could learn the skills privately. This outraged many in the industry—they didn't like their secrets being told, and they ostracized Spaulding for selling equipment to the general public. But love them or hate them, Huck Spaulding and his supply partner, Paul Rogers, were a huge influence on the evolution of tattoo art.

The downside of that contribution, however, was the introduction of "scratchers." These are the people who know just enough about tattooing to be dangerous. They buy the supplies, but they don't bother to sterilize them and often don't even know how. They "scratch" their friends, causing irreversible damage through scarring or the spread of infection and disease. Indeed, it's a slippery slope: The more readily available the equipment is and the more of a moneymaking opportunity tattooing becomes, the more scratchers emerge.

But the easy access to equipment wasn't all bad. Soon, the term "self-taught" was being used by many promising artists, thanks to the running start provided by Spaulding and Rogers. Since there wasn't any serious investment required, many contemporary artists tried their hand at this new medium, inadvertently merging styles and creating a whole new genre.

I entered the tattoo world in 1996, and I've seen a lot of changes even since then. I've seen hundreds of scratchers arrested for illegal tattooing; I've witnessed the lifting of almost every major tattoo ban—New York City, Norfolk, Massachusetts, South Carolina, and Oklahoma; I've seen the increase in companies who've become tattoo-friendly instead of discriminating.

The current generation of tattoo artists is a completely different breed from that which started it all. The old-timers would say that tattooing has lost some of its charm, while the new-schoolers would argue that progress is good. Either way, both generations have contributed to the current mainstream popularity of what was once considered taboo.

TIP: There's some conjecture about where body art is heading. In another twenty to thirty years, the currently modified masses will be past or approaching middle age. I'd like to think that we're heading toward equality for all with tattoos and body piercings, especially in the workplace. When the conservative generations are no longer in charge of big business, a more accepting and open group of people will take over. Will we see the day when even the president is tattooed and pierced? Hey, it could happen!

who gets tattoos and why?

> *"When I first got my gay pride tat, it was because I was kinda cocky and wanted it to be an 'in your face' kinda thing. It eventually turned into more than that. It has become a part of me—a symbol of who I am and of the fight that gay women and men go through to have the same rights as others. I don't even show it much anymore, because it's more personal to me now."*
>
> **— STACEY**

You may not be shocked when you see tattoos on bikers, military personnel, or people who work in tattoo shops. But you might be very surprised to know how many tattoos are hiding under fancy suits, doctors' cloaks, and teachers' dresses. These days, people from all walks of life are getting marked for life. Some of them may have very small designs that are easy to obscure, but a tattoo is still a tattoo, and more and more people are getting them.

So why do people get them? There are so many reasons; theoretically, almost everyone could have a different reason to ink themselves.

✑ Personal or Religious Rites

Although ritualistic tattooing is ancient history for many of us in Western society, rite-of-passage tattooing does still exist. These deeply rooted traditions are essential to many cultures, marking a significant point in one's life, such as ascension into adulthood or achieving a certain level of honor.

✑ Personal Expression

This is probably the most common reason people get tattooed. It's a way to represent yourself in an artistic and creative way that separates you from everyone else. Even though the person standing next to you may also have tattoos, the pictures and placement will be different, thus creating a very personal identity. You might get tattoos that symbolize your tastes in music, hobbies, or sports teams, or something that expresses what you feel inside. They say "a picture is worth a thousand words," and a person covered with tattoos is a veritable book of information without ever having to open their mouth.

✑ In Honor of or in Memoriam

Another top reason people get tattoos, even if they never thought of having one before, is to honor someone they love. Getting a tattoo in honor of someone, whether living or dead, seems to be the ultimate sign of devotion. Many people say that the emotional pain from losing a loved one is eased through the physical pain of getting a tattoo.

✑ Political or Personal Statements

Getting a tattoo that represents something you care about deeply is a powerful way to share your view with the world. Supporting certain rights or championing a cause is often a big enough reason to be inked for life.

Marking a Significant Event or Life Change

Sometimes circling a date on a calendar just doesn't cut it. Surviving cancer, the birth of a child, celebrating sobriety, and coming out are just some of the many reasons people choose to mark a date or event with a permanent reminder.

Permanent Cosmetics

Permanent cosmetics are not just for vanity purposes, although they certainly can make applying daily makeup much less work! Cosmetic tattoos have answered the prayers of many battling alopecia (loss of hair, including eyelashes and eyebrows) and vitiligo (loss of skin pigmentation). Women who have had breast reconstruction after a mastectomy can get areola repigmentation, and some women simply choose to have a beautiful design tattooed over their scars, rather than opting for reconstruction.

Artistic Interest

Some people get tattooed simply because they like the way tattoos look. They choose designs that have artistic value—sometimes patterns or pictures that follow a theme. There's absolutely nothing wrong with getting a tattoo "just because," as long as you're sure it's something you'll continue to enjoy for the rest of your life.

Rebellion

Although it may not be the wisest reason to get a tattoo, I suppose there's always a slight feeling of rebellion in all of us when we get inked. But some people get a tattoo to rebel against society, or even to rebel against a specific person, like a parent. Unfortunately, these are the tattoos that usually turn into a regret at some point down the road.

ೋ Social Acceptance

Getting a tattoo simply "because everyone else has one" is probably the worst reason to do so. But, inevitably, there are those who will do so to fit in, to be cool, to imitate their favorite pop star, or for whatever other reason that has nothing to do with a sincere personal desire to be inked. You should never (never!) feel pressured to get a tattoo if it's not something you really want for yourself.

fear and pain

Although tattoos are completely voluntary, it's normal to experience anxiety. Lots of people are able to shake it off and go forward with their decision, but others are held back by their fears. If you're afraid of pain, needles, blood, or simply the unknown, you're not alone! This chapter will empower you with the knowledge you need to make your foray into the world of body art an exciting and *positive* experience.

What does it feel like to get a tattoo? Does it hurt? Well, yes—to be truthful, it does. But then again, so does stubbing your toe, and I'd much rather get a tattoo than jam my toe against the bedpost. But stubbing your toe isn't crippling or traumatic—and neither is getting a tattoo.

Granted, some areas of the body are more tender and sensitive to pain than others. You may hear some people say not to get a tattoo on the ankle or wrist because it hurts more when it's close to bone. That is actually a myth. While the ankle and wrist certainly are more tender, it's because of the skin, not its close vicinity to bone. The skin in these locations—as well as the skin on the neck, under the arms, and in the sternum and/

or breast regions—is thinner and has nerves very close to the surface. Breaking through these softer zones and into sensitive nerves is bound to cause more pain than breaking the skin on the back, upper arm, or thigh, where the skin is thicker.

When the tattoo needles first touch your skin, it's uncomfortable. It feels a bit like being scratched by a cat or stung by a bee—sharp and hot at the same time. The needles move up and down so fast, however, that you don't actually feel each individual poke. But you do feel *something*, and the longer the line the artist has to draw without stopping, the more irritating the sensation. That's how most people would describe the overall feeling of getting tattooed—annoying. Throughout the course of getting the tattoo, you may wince or clench your teeth, but that's usually the most severe reaction.

So then why do you hear stories about people crying or passing out from getting tattooed? Granted, some people are more sensitive than others, but a lot of people assume they're the sensitive type and have a low pain tolerance. It's very, very rare that a person is so sensitive that it makes them cry. When this happens, there's a good chance their body was overly stressed to begin with, or maybe they were overly sensitive and really weren't able to handle the pain.

If your body is already under some kind of strain—whether it is a physical illness, your menstrual cycle, or emotional stress—it may be wise to put off getting a tattoo. Your tolerance for pain is diminished when your body is already compromised from trying to deal with something else. This is why it's not recommended that you get a tattoo when you have a cold; or if it's been less than six weeks since giving birth or having some type of surgery or dental work; or if you've been in a minor accident. These are the kinds of things that drain your body of its pain- and infection-fighting resources. It's always best to wait until you're completely recovered before making your tattoo appointment.

By the way, fainting isn't a symptom of pain. It results from a severe drop in blood sugar, which can be brought on by anxiety or not eating.

Therefore, it's really important to eat a healthy snack or small meal about an hour before you get a tattoo, and try not to get yourself too worked up about it. When under stress or in pain, the body releases adrenaline. The "letdown" from discovering that the process isn't nearly as painful as anticipated can cause the body to realize it has an overabundance of adrenaline, which can lead to lightheadedness or fainting. If you do feel faint during a session, tell your artist. Most likely, they'll stop and offer you a cool towel or a piece of candy to boost your blood sugar. Usually, that's all it takes before you're feeling just fine again.

The use of numbing creams, such as EMLA or lidocaine, is not endorsed by most artists. First of all, they have to be prescribed by a physician and used under a physician's supervision. Second, they take over half an hour to take effect, and then numb the pain only minimally and temporarily. The returning sensation when the numbing wears off is sometimes worse than the original pain would've been—which, as I've said, usually isn't that bad. Most artists consider numbing creams more trouble than they're worth, but if you're really set on the idea of using one, you can talk to your artist and doctor and see if something can be worked out.

The best way to deal with fear and/or anxiety is distraction. Bring a friend with you to hold your hand. Listen to music, chew gum, read a magazine, or talk with the artist. Find other things to focus on—like how cool your tattoo is going to look when it's finished!

✆ Get That Needle Away from Me!

Fear of needles and fear of blood are bigger obstacles than fear of pain. I can assure you that the pain isn't going to be that bad, but I can't cure you of a deeply rooted associative fear. However, knowledge is power, and it may help you to know a few things before entering the tattoo studio.

When we think of needles, we usually think of the hypodermic syringes that nurses use to give a shot. I don't like those kinds of needles any more than the next person, but tattoo needles are quite different. Understanding the differences may help you overcome your fear.

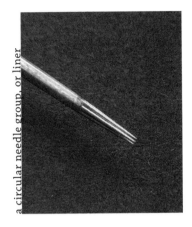

a circular needle group, or liner

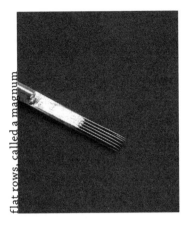

flat rows, called a magnum

Tattoo needles, called sharps, are very similar to stickpins in size. You're usually tattooed with not just one tattoo sharp, but several soldered together; this is called a needle group. A needle group can consist of anywhere between three and fifteen sharps (sometimes more) and can be shaped into a circle or flat rows. Circular needle groups are generally used for outlining and are called liners. Needle groups of two or more flat rows are called magnums (or mags) and are generally used for shading. The idea of so many needles may make you shudder, but think of it this way: When a sideshow performer lies down on a bed of nails, the reason they don't impale him is because more nails means a better ratio of skin to spikes. In the same way, more needles in a needle group actually causes less pain; plus, it helps the artist get the job done more quickly, which means you get out of the chair sooner.

Another difference between tattoo needles and syringes is how deeply they penetrate the skin. A tattoo needle seeks to only break the surface of the skin to implant the ink underneath the uppermost layers. Ever get a paper cut? A tattoo needle doesn't go any farther than that. Sure, it's a little painful, but certainly nothing you can't endure.

❧ Don't Look Down!

If you're afraid of seeing blood, you'll hopefully be encouraged by this news: Most tattoos produce only a few drops of blood, and some produce none at all. For those few drops that your tattoo might create, it would be advisable to turn your head until your artist has had time to clean it up. Larger tattoos can bleed more, but there are things you can do to reduce the amount of blood loss during the procedure. (Read more about this in Chapter 15.)

If you simply can't bear to watch the procedure but still really want a tattoo, my only suggestion is that you get the tattoo in an area where you can't watch, or wear a blindfold. But if your fear is severe, think twice before making an appointment. Trust me, you don't want to freak out on your artist. (Chances are they are booked solid and don't have the time or the inclination to deal with high-maintenance clients. Frankly, that's not their job.) Master yourself and see it as a challenge to be conquered—or simply don't get tattooed.

Remember, the point of getting a tattoo is that it's something that you *really* want. If that's the case, go for it. If you're going to let excuses get in your way, then something is telling you that a tattoo is not right for you—at least not yet. Don't let anyone, including yourself, pressure you into getting one if it's not something you truly desire. A tattoo is a lifelong commitment and should never be gotten on a whim or a dare, or out of some sense of obligation.

permanence
and commitment

With all types of body art, there's a level of commitment that goes along with them, and tattoos are one of the most permanent forms of body art. The ink gets injected about one or two millimeters under the skin, which doesn't seem like much, but it's enough to make the ink become a part of your body as it heals. Sure, you can have it removed with laser treatments if you're really not happy with it, but that's a complicated and painful (not to mention expensive!) procedure that can leave scars behind.

✎ Magic Disappearing Ink?

You may have heard a lot of press hype in recent years about "smart tattoos" and "disappearing ink." This refers to a new type of tattoo ink that has been developed using a technology created by Brown University scientist Edith Mathiowitz. Mathiowitz developed a microcapsule delivery system for medication, but has been working with Freedom2, Inc., to encapsulate tattoo inks instead of drugs. The premise is that the tiny polymer beads protect the body from any toxins contained in the ink and make removing the tattoo easier because those little beads are easily burst with a laser, and then the ink is simply washed away by the body's own natural defenses. While it's easy to get excited by anything with a space-age-sounding technology, so far these inks have fallen short of expectations. There are very few colors available, and the end results are not impressive. The colors are muted and don't offer the smoothness and depth of traditional tattoo inks. To be honest, a real tattoo artist will have no use for this kind of ink, or a client that is so unsure about their desire to get a tattoo that they would even request it.

⁓ No Cold Feet Allowed

For serious collectors, part of the attraction of getting a tattoo is the permanence. It's a commitment, and one willingly made by those who have that deep connection with the art. Do you have that level of respect for the tattoo you are considering getting?

The type of tattoo you choose to get can affect your chances of regret at some point in life. See Chapter 11, "Choosing and Creating Your Design," to see what kinds of tattoos tend to result in the greatest number of removals and cover-ups.

TIP: You can temporarily cover a tattoo if you need to conceal it for a few hours, such as for a wedding or other special occasion. High-end department stores sell cover-up makeup, like Dermablend, that is very opaque and can effectively conceal tattoos. There are also a couple of products available online, such as Tattoo Camo and ColorTration, that come in different shades to better match your personal skin tone; stage/theater makeup (e.g., Ben Nye) also works well. Airbrushing not only covers well, but has more staying power than makeup. So, even though the tattoo is permanent, there are ways to camouflage it short-term.

religious, social, and employment conflicts

Wanting a tattoo and being a member of a religion or church that frowns upon them can be a difficult personal struggle. Many Christian sects and the Jewish faith refer to a scripture from the Old Testament (Leviticus 19:28) that states, "Ye shall not make any cuttings in your flesh for the dead, nor print any marks upon you: I am the LORD." According to this Bible verse, it does sound quite plain that printing marks upon your flesh—i.e., tattoos—would be a direct sin.

The problem, though, with taking any one verse from the Bible and using it as a stand-alone directive is the way in which everything else around it is ignored or forgotten. There are many directives given in the Old Testament that Christians do not follow. Otherwise, eating pork or shellfish, cutting your hair, or wearing clothing woven from two different fabrics would be as sinful as getting a tattoo.

Many Christians and Jews have tattoos, and a lot of them get them to signify their faiths—crosses and portraits of Jesus Christ are among some of the most popular tattoo icons.

Orthodox Jews expressly forbid tattoos, but even those among their ranks have been known to get inked, and oftentimes also choose tattoos that show pride in their faith. You may have heard that if a Jew has a tattoo, they can't be buried in a Jewish cemetery when they die. Turns out, that old edict is a myth; it was probably a rumor started many years ago as a way to dissuade Jews from getting inked. It's understandable, considering the stigmatic relationship between Jews and tattoos because of the way permanent marks were forced on them during the Holocaust, but the "no Jewish burial" claims simply aren't true. Rabbi Barton Lee from Arizona State University Hillel states, "Their folks aren't going to like this, but they're wrong." Since his proclamation, several other rabbis have come forward to dispel the myth about Jews, tattoos, and burial rites, although many of them still feel that getting inked goes against their basic beliefs.

Islam, one of the stricter faiths, especially where matters of vanity or personal decoration are concerned, teaches that getting a tattoo destroys one's relationship with God. That's a very serious consequence. And yet many Muslims have joined the ranks of the inked.

So, since tattoos are present even among members of religions that forbid them, does that mean it's okay for you to get one if you're a member of one of these faiths?

That's a very personal decision, and one that I can't make for you. However, my thoughts on the matter are these: If you think getting a tattoo will, in any way, make you stumble in your faith or harm your relationship with God, then you shouldn't do it. If it could cause others around you in your faith to stumble, then you should seriously consider that first. But if you feel secure in your faith and you choose a tattoo that isn't offensive or hurtful to anyone, then that is between you and God. No one has the right to judge you for your decision.

∝ Family and Social Conflicts

Even if your religion doesn't tell you that you can't get a tattoo, your family and friends might. Disapproval from those around us can vary from being a simple look of disappointment to being total ostracism. It's hard to believe a picture on the skin can cause such a stir of emotions, but some people really take offense to the idea.

If you know that people in your family or social circles have a problem with tattoos, you need to recognize the fact that you might become a victim of discrimination from those you feel closest to. That kind of prejudice is even harder to take than that of strangers.

If you know that getting inked is going to be a sensitive issue, it's best not to show up at a family or social gathering, pull up your sleeve, and say, "Surprise!" Just like with any other controversial subject, it's better to speak to the potentially offended person or persons privately and explain your reasons for getting tattooed. It's always possible that you may even be able to win them over by showing your concern for their feelings in the matter. And then again, it may not go over well at all, and you will simply have to give it time and hope they eventually come around.

Sometimes the circumstances surrounding the choice of getting tattooed are even more serious than disapproval. Some parents have threatened to cut off college funding for children if they dare to be inked. One mother even refused to go to her daughter's wedding if she didn't find a way to "cover up that hideous thing." This is when it becomes a much larger issue and may even require putting off getting tattooed at all or finding a very effective way to keep it hidden!

✍ Employment Issues

It's difficult enough finding a good job these days, and unfortunately, no matter how many degrees you have or how well you're trained, tattoos will turn off the average white-collar employer in a heartbeat. Even many blue-collar and entry-level jobs are open only to people without visible tattoos (or piercings). Unmodified people are getting harder to find as body art becomes more popular, but the majority of employers refuse to yield to its growing acceptability.

If you have lofty goals for your future, visible tattoos are going to hinder your progress. It's not right, it's not fair, but it's fact. If you're planning on going into a field where you'll be wearing a suit all the time, you have more options since the suit will cover most of your body. But if the job doesn't require a suit, and you don't want to be stuck wearing long sleeves every day for the rest of your life, you need to think carefully before getting inked on your arms, chest, calves, and other highly visible areas.

Even if you're currently in a job that is more laid-back and your boss has never had a problem with your tattoos, keep in mind that things could change. A new boss could come in, or you could be laid off and forced to find new employment, and the tattoos would suddenly become an issue again. Because tattoos are permanent and still controversial, you have to consider your future many years down the road before making the commitment to get inked, especially in a noticeable area of your body.

I'd be the last person to dissuade someone from getting inked if it's something they really want, but I think having a good job, having goals, and being an asset to society are more important than a tattoo. Making a personal compromise to get a tattoo in a place that's easy to keep covered is a reasonable trade-off if it means it won't hurt your ability to attain your goals in life.

health issues and blood donation

∽ Preexisting Health Issues

A new tattoo is an open wound. Your body needs to be able to stop bleeding, fight infection, and heal itself after the procedure. Diseases that lower your body's ability to do these things can make getting a tattoo life-threatening. When you're faced with a choice between your health and a tattoo, I certainly hope that you will choose your health.

If you have a preexisting health issue that compromises your immune system or makes it difficult to heal wounds—such as HIV or diabetes—getting a tattoo is a much greater risk than it would be for someone with a clean bill of health. That doesn't mean you can't get a tattoo, but it does mean you have to take your decision much more seriously than other people, and that you need to recognize the dangers involved.

HIV and hepatitis seriously compromise the body's immune system and make it difficult to fight off infection. Most tattoos don't run the risk of infection, but it can happen. Staph infections, in particular, are a big risk, even in very clean situations. A staph infection can take down a normally healthy person; its effects on someone who's already weakened can be deadly. If you have a disease that causes a lowered immune response, you should ask your doctor first before getting a tattoo.

You may not think of diabetes as a serious disease in comparison with HIV, but it also jeopardizes the body's ability to heal. Small scratches and wounds that would be little more than an annoyance to most of us can result in days or weeks of painful recovery for a diabetic. Only those who have their blood sugar under control should even consider getting a tattoo, and even then they should do so under the advisement of their doctor or endocrinologist.

Getting a tattoo can also be extremely dangerous for hemophiliacs. Although tattoo needles don't penetrate the skin very deeply, they do draw blood. An inability to stop the bleeding could land you in the hospital. On a side note, a tattoo that won't stop bleeding can flush out too much ink and leave you with an ugly, splotchy picture.

A weak heart is another dangerous condition when it comes to getting a tattoo, even if you are taking medication for it. Young people, especially, ignore this risk, and several have died because of it. Talk with your doctor, and don't be surprised if they advise against getting a tattoo. Again, please choose your health above all else.

Even if your doctor says "not now," that doesn't mean "not ever." Maybe right now your body isn't able to heal a tattoo properly, but in the coming weeks or months, by taking care of yourself, following your treatment regimen, or even simply waiting for a time when your body is stronger, a tattoo may still be a possibility.

↶ Full Disclosure

If you do have a disease or health issue that could affect your ability to be tattooed safely, it is extremely important that you be honest with your tattoo artist about it. Most release forms you sign before getting inked ask clearly if you have any communicable diseases or a compromised immune system, or if you feel there is any reason a tattoo could put you at risk. You must answer this honestly! If you don't, you could be putting yourself or your artist in unnecessary danger.

∽ Communicable Diseases

If you have a communicable disease like HIV or hepatitis, don't assume that a tattoo artist will turn you away if you tell them. Professional tattoo artists follow Standard Precautions, which are specific safety measures that are designated by the Centers for Disease Control and Prevention (CDC) to reduce the risk of disease exposure from blood and/or bodily fluids. As part of the Standard Precautions training, artists treat every customer as if they have a communicable disease. So if you actually have one, it shouldn't change anything for them. But it does help for them to be aware of the situation and also helps them serve you better as artists. They'll know your body has a difficult time fighting infection, so they will work even harder to keep you safe and coach you in proper aftercare that will give you the best chance of an uneventful recovery.

In the event that an artist does turn you away, you may have legal recourse, depending on where you live and what your local discrimination laws are. But honestly, you're better off just letting it go and finding someone else to work on you. These unprofessional tattooers do exist, but they're few and far between.

∽ Blood Donation Restriction

If you are healthy and choose to get a tattoo, you still need to realize that there are some self-imposed restrictions you subject yourself to. The main one is your ability to donate blood or plasma.

Although the American Red Cross has been making some changes to these laws due to the lack of qualified donors, in most places you still have to wait a year after being tattooed to donate blood or plasma. This is to reduce your risk of spreading disease that may have been contracted during the procedure.

In states that have strict regulations—meaning the health

department dictates how a tattoo shop should run and conducts regular inspections to be sure it's running properly—you are allowed to donate blood as long as you can prove that you received your tattoo at a licensed shop in that state. Otherwise, you are still subject to the one-year wait, even if you got it at a perfectly safe or licensed shop in another state.

Blood donation is an important and honorable thing to do, and having to wait an entire year to donate can be a big deal if it's something you normally do regularly. In the United States, you can donate blood about six times a year, plasma up to twelve times a year. That's a lot of people you can potentially help by being able to continue donating. If giving the gift of life through blood donation is important to you, then you need to take this into consideration before getting a tattoo.

body issues

Every human body is different from the next, which means that no two tattoos—even identical designs—are exactly alike. Body chemistry, differences in skin tone, and even your current health affect how well a tattoo will take and heal. Future changes to your body can also affect how your tattoo will age over the years. All these things need to be taken into consideration before and after you get inked.

✐ Weight Fluctuation

Most of us deal with minor ups and downs in body weight as we age and go through different stages of life. Slight changes in body size will have little effect on a tattoo, but major weight gain or loss can distort a tattoo image.

Pregnancy is the most common quick-onset weight gain and loss that can result in major body-shape changes. If a tattoo happens to be on a part of the body where the skin will be stretching, then it is possible that your tattoo will be stretched into an abnormal shape. Like a woman's belly, a design can also make a full recovery, but this depends on the elasticity of the skin, whether any stretch marks develop on the tattoo itself, and whether the body actually goes back to the way it was before pregnancy. Because of the high level of risk of damaging a tattoo as a result of pregnancy, I usually recommend that women of childbearing age avoid getting inked in the stomach or abdominal regions.

Any significant weight loss or gain has the potential to change the appearance of a tattoo. But overall body weight gain—unlike pregnancy—poses much less risk in that regard. These changes are usually made more slowly, giving the skin time to adjust. Even fifty pounds of weight gain or loss is going to change the diameter of an arm or a leg by only a few inches—not enough to significantly change the overall appearance of a tattoo. But there are exceptions—for instance, when dealing with an intricately detailed tattoo. With significant weight gain, the lines may spread out, and much of the detail can be lost or turn fuzzy. With significant weight loss, those already small lines will squish together and could turn details into a blob.

Another exception involves those tattoos with specific shapes, like circles, squares, and other forms with definite structural attributes, which are at significant risk for distortion if there is a substantial change in body size or shape.

✧ Stretch Marks

Stretch marks, or striae, which are actually a type of scar, are probably the most damaging results of weight gain (or sometimes even drastic weight loss). They appear as narrow grooves or channels in the skin and are caused by more stress on the skin than its natural elasticity will allow. When that happens, the dermis (middle layer) of skin actually tears, and sometimes tiny capillaries and blood vessels are broken and blood is released into the tissue, causing a red or purple hue. As they heal, some stretch marks appear flush to the skin and light in color, while others can remain deeper and much more severe.

If striae happen to form through a preexisting tattoo, they could cause permanent damage to the art. If a stretch mark is faint and not deep,

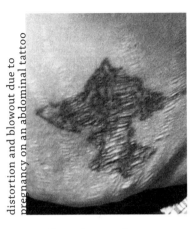

rejected navel piercing scar and ink blowout due to pregnancy

distortion and blowout due to pregnancy on an abdominal tattoo

it won't distort the overall image, but the odds of the scar disappearing and the tattoo actually going back to normal are very slim. If you develop a deep, dark stretch mark through your ink, there is almost no chance of recovery. The reason stretch marks sometimes appear lighter than your natural skin color after they have healed is because natural pigmentation is lost in that area of damaged skin, and it's difficult to predict what it will do to artificial pigmentation from a tattoo.

It is possible, however, to tattoo over preexisting stretch marks, especially light or superficial marks. Deep or dark ones pose a bigger problem and aren't as effectively covered with ink. The light stretch marks I have on the underside of my arm practically disappeared when I had them tattooed. It's a very effective way to beautify something you may feel self-conscious about.

∽ Injury, Surgery, and Scars (Oh My!)

What happens if you sustain a serious injury in the area of your tattoo, or if you're required to have surgery that cuts through your tattoo? In most cases, the damage done to the tattoo is irreparable. The best way to handle this is to have the area covered up with a new design once the wound is healed.

If there is any raised scarring, allow extra healing time (even as much as two years) for the tissue to soften and blend better with the skin before trying to tattoo over it. Vitamin E helps to make scarring more supple and will aid the healing process. Many scars can be tattooed very effectively, and some will refuse to hold ink no matter what you do. If you have some scarring you'd like to try to tattoo over, consult with your artist and see if they think it's worth a shot. If not, scars can also be worked into a design, so you may just have to get creative!

౼ Skin Issues

Skin conditions, such as acne, psoriasis, and eczema, need special consideration before you get a tattoo, as do skin growths, such as moles and cysts. Blemishes and abnormalities on the skin can affect your ability to be tattooed effectively or safely.

ACNE

If you want to get tattooed in an area you tend to break out in, make sure you wait until the breakout subsides before getting inked. However, if you're prone to regular acne breakouts in the region you want tattooed, those pustules and the resulting scars can really mess up your artwork, and I would recommend against getting tattooed there. (See also Chapter 15, "Food, Drink, Medication, and Drugs," if you are currently taking prescription medication for acne.)

PSORIASIS

Although there are several types of psoriasis, it generally affects the surface of the skin in the form of inflammation, scaly patches (plaque), or pustules. The disease can range in severity from mild to acute and is treated in many different ways. Depending on your particular case, it may or may not be advisable to get a tattoo, and this is something you should first discuss with your attending physician. But any damage to the skin (on a person who already suffers from psoriasis) can result in what is called the Koebner effect. That means an area of skin previously unaffected by psoriasis could form new lesions due to trauma from a scratch or puncture.

Not every psoriasis sufferer is prone to the Koebner effect, and even those who are can sometimes be successfully tattooed with no ill effects. However, there are also those who have either gotten new plaque from a tattoo or had their condition spread to—and thus damage—their artwork. There are a rare few who have actually reported improvement in their skin health after getting a tattoo, although there doesn't seem to be any rationale or proof behind these claims.

Needless to say, most artists will not tattoo anywhere that is actively broken out with psoriasis, and you should carefully consider whether you should get a tattoo if you have this condition.

ECZEMA

Also a condition of the skin, eczema (or atopic dermatitis) is actually an allergic condition that can be triggered by many elements. People with eczema experience red, swollen, itchy rashes as a result of exposure to a variety of allergens, environmental conditions, and even stress. Because eczema sufferers can get flare-ups from unknown substances, it is generally inadvisable to get a tattoo. There's no telling how your body is going to react to the ink, and unfortunately—because ink makers are not required by law to make their ingredients publicly available—it's difficult to know exactly what you might be introducing into your body that could trigger a reaction. But it never hurts to discuss the possibility with your doctor. If your condition is mild, your doctor may feel your personal risk is minimal.

SKIN GROWTHS

There are many types of growths that can affect the skin, most of which are benign, but what should you do if you have one of these growths in the same area where you are planning to be tattooed?

As a general rule, moles, cysts, lipomas, granulomas, fibromas, and most other skin growths should not be tattooed. They can be tattooed around, but the growths should be left alone. Although your cyst or mole may never be anything more than that, it should be treated as an indicator of possible trouble. These growths will change in size, color, or shape if they become malignant (or cancerous), and tattooing over them could result in your missing a very important sign of change.

In the event that your doctor needed to perform a biopsy or even remove cancerous cells, it would damage your tattoo anyway, so it's just not a great idea to get tattooed anywhere you may be at risk for cancerous development.

Keloids should not be tattooed, and those prone to keloiding may want to avoid getting tattooed altogether. For more information on this, see Chapter 22, "Troubleshooting Tattoo Problems."

Freckles, on the other hand, are the only skin condition that does not pose any danger. Even if some of your freckles are slightly raised, they should not prevent you from getting tattooed. But keep in mind that tattoo ink does not completely cover freckles, so some of them may still show through, especially through light or bright colors.

scratchers versus professionals

When you see your doctor, you know that they've had to successfully complete their medical training and obtain proper degrees, licensing, and credentials in order to practice. Not so with a tattoo artist.

While some states require licensing of a studio, individual artists do not necessarily have to be licensed or certified. And anyone can start tattooing out of their home, whether it's legal or not—tattooing equipment and supplies are readily available to the general public. There are a staggering number of people tattooing out of their kitchens, basements, and garages, and they have absolutely no formal training or any regard for cleanliness and sterility. These people are called "scratchers." Scratchers, kitchen magicians, basement butchers—whatever you prefer, these names speak to the subpar quality of their services and the poor conditions under which they work. Let's compare the specific differences between a scratcher and a professional tattoo artist.

∽ Tools of the Trade

Professional tattoo artists have access to the best equipment in the business and will buy what they feel gives them an edge in the quality of their artwork.

They buy machines that run smoothly, making the experience of getting tattooed less painful and less damaging to the skin. They buy high-quality needles, which are sharp and precise and provide the best ink delivery for your tattoo. They use high-quality inks, which contain safe ingredients and give the best and brightest color results possible.

Scratchers buy the cheapest machine they can buy or, worse, use some kind of handmade device with a motor stolen from an electric razor or a pencil sharpener. The needles, if they're using actual needles, are mass-produced, and the sharps are not precisely lined, which means more pain and more skin damage. Some of them still have flux residue on them, which is extremely dangerous and can cause infection. Of course, there are those who prefer to use sewing needles or guitar strings—even better! And ink? If you're lucky, they're using some of the cheaply made tattoo inks, which are at least usually safe but produce really lousy color results. A lot of kitchen magicians, however, prefer the more economical and readily available India ink, or printer ink. On the worst end of the spectrum are those creative former convicts who know how to mix their own special brew using cigarette ashes and metal filings with a little fruit juice and saliva mixed in. Now, doesn't that sound lovely?

∽ Talent and Quality

A professional tattoo artist must have at least some talent, or he/she wouldn't have been hired to work in a professional studio. Granted, some have more than others. Some artists have natural talent they've developed to create incredible tattoo art. Some of them even have formal art training and a college degree in fine arts. And all of them have a portfolio at the shop that shows you exactly how qualified they are and what they are capable of.

Scratchers may or may not have talent. Most of them are working out of their home because they're in it only to make money. People willing to give them business usually aren't looking for fine art or high quality— they're looking for a cheap tattoo. There is always the rare case of someone

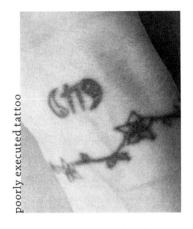

poorly executed tattoo

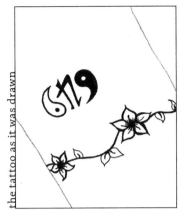

the tattoo as it was drawn

who really has a talent for the art and has simply taken the wrong path. But what the patrons of these scratchers don't realize is that along with that cheap tattoo, they might be taking home a disease as well.

Cleanliness Isn't Just for Appearances

Cleanliness is the main difference between a scratcher and a professional. A professional has access to an ultrasonic sanitizer, which removes particles of ink and blood from metal tattooing equipment. Afterward, each piece is placed in a sterilizing pouch and then in an autoclave sterilizer, which is a very expensive piece of equipment that kills bacteria and blood-borne pathogens on all metal equipment that is reused from client to client.

But that's just the beginning. Professional artists properly sanitize their stations between clients; they use plastic barriers on lamps, phones, and other things they have to touch, so as not to spread disease; they protect the items that can't be autoclaved—such as their tattoo machines, clip cords, and spray bottles—with plastic; they wear gloves and change them frequently to prevent cross-contamination. Most important, they practice these safe methods—named Standard Precautions by the CDC— on each and every client, doing everything they can to provide the client with the cleanest and safest experience possible.

Scratchers, on the other hand, will try to give the appearance of cleanliness. They may wear gloves, but they touch and cross-contaminate everything they come in contact with. They won't use an autoclave sterilizer, but they'll assure you that the pressure cooker they use on their kitchen stove is just as effective. Of course, some don't even bother to use a pressure cooker, and will insist that boiling the needles and tubes kills the germs. And then there are the really safety-conscious scratchers who just wipe everything off with a strong antibacterial cleaning solution. Some buy single-use needles and tubes, but if they don't know how to clean and sanitize their other equipment, you're still at risk of coming in contact with bacteria or a disease.

It's pretty obvious that most of us would rather go to the clean, safe studio with an experienced and clean artist who can ensure a safe tattoo experience and a beautiful piece of art than to the kitchen magician with a homemade tattoo machine and unknown ink ingredients. But it doesn't always work out that way. Sometimes the opportunity for a cheap tattoo is just too tempting when you're partying with friends or know someone trying to self-teach who offers to practice on you for free. Young people are lured in by the chance to skirt the law a bit and get a tattoo without having to wait until they're legally of age. Honestly, though, if you choose to go with a scratcher, don't be surprised if you end up regretting your tattoo somewhere down the road. I have several artist friends in the business who do just as much cover-up work as they do new tattoos.

I worked with a lady several years ago who had a homemade flower (at least I think it was supposed to be a flower) tattoo on her arm. It was so poorly done, and she was embarrassed by it. She wore long sleeves on hot days just to keep it covered, and if people happened to get a glimpse of it and ask about it, she would lower her head and shyly explain that she didn't like it and wanted to get it removed. One crappy tattoo caused that woman pain, not just a mild case of regret. Tattoos become such a part of your skin and body that a bad one can feel like an ugly physical flaw.

touring the studio

A tattoo studio is a unique place when it comes to the stuff you'll see, hear, and smell. Some find tattoo shops to be inviting and wonderful places. Aside from the few shops that still live up to the "seedy dive" stereotype, most are cleaner than your average doctor's office. One of the first things you'll see when you enter a tattoo shop is the flash displays. Flash is the name for the sheets of predrawn art you see hanging on walls, in racks, or in binders at most tattoo shops. Studios that do only custom artwork usually do not display flash art. It exists for customers to peruse and get a taste for the kind of work that's done at the studio—even if you already know what tattoo you're going to get.

The sounds associated with a tattoo shop are also wholly their own. Many studios will have music playing in the background, but the style and volume of that music can be very diverse from shop to shop. But there's one constant: the buzz of the tattoo machine.

❧ Buzz, Buzz, Buzz

The most common sound heard in a tattoo shop is that of an active tattoo machine. It makes a rather loud vibrating sound, similar to an electric shaver's. Some find the buzzing of a tattoo machine melodic or entrancing, while others find it irritating or grating, like a dentist's drill. If you happen to be someone who doesn't enjoy the sound of a tattoo machine, you might want to bring your MP3 player with you.

❧ How a Tattoo Machine Works

The tattoo machine is a relatively simple, but beautiful and highly respected, tool of the trade. It consists of a power supply, a foot switch, electromagnets, a spring-loaded metal arm, a hollow grip tube, and a needle—or cluster of needles—on the end of a long metal bar (needle bar). The power supply allows the artist to adjust the voltage that is sent to the tattoo machine. When the tattoo artist steps on the foot switch, electricity is fed to the tattoo machine through the electromagnetic coils. But if that electrical current were steady, the needle would just sit there, like a click pen with the pen tip stuck in the "out" position. So, in order to create the up-and-down motion, the electrical current is temporarily interrupted, which releases the needle back to its original position inside the grip tube. When that happens, the electrical current is activated once again, pushing the needle back down. As difficult as it is to imagine, this happens over a hundred times per second—the needle movement is so fast, it's not visible to the human eye; instead it just looks like the tip of the needle is vibrating. It's a lot like a sewing machine, except that the range of motion is much, much shorter since the tattoo needle moves only a fraction of an inch.

The tattoo needle moves inside a barrel-shaped tube that keeps the motion straight. When the artist dips the needle into the ink, it grabs a small droplet and pulls it up into the tip of the tube, which serves as a reservoir. A small droplet of ink can actually last several rounds of needle penetration. When the supply runs low, the artist simply dips the needles back into the ink for more.

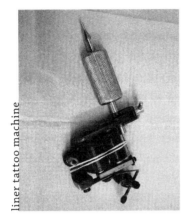

liner tattoo machine

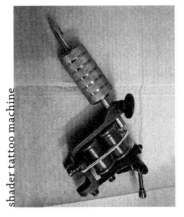

shader tattoo machine

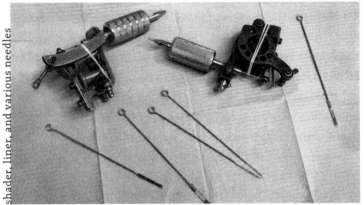

shader, liner, and various needles

TIP: Don't ever refer to a tattoo machine as a "gun." It's an offensive term to most professionals because it's the preferred term used by scratchers. Since the tattoo machine is the very heart and soul of the trade, it deserves much respect.

ASSESSING YOUR FIRST IMPRESSIONS

When you first walk into a tattoo studio, the entrance area should be neat, clean, and welcoming. Most have chairs for waiting clients to sit on.

Are they clean and well maintained, or dirty and tattered? If there is a fish tank, do the fish look well cared for, and is the water clean? Does the floor look like it's mopped or vacuumed regularly? Do you smell cigarette smoke? Smoking in the shop is a huge no-no! The first few minutes you spend in a tattoo studio can tell you a lot about how the rest of it—and its clients—are cared for.

Once you've entered the shop, you should be greeted by an employee. Some studios don't have a receptionist, and it can be difficult for the artists to get up in the middle of doing a tattoo to greet a newcomer. If this is the case, the artists should be easily accessible, or even viewable, from their stations. You shouldn't have to wait around too long before someone comes to talk to you, even if they ask you to come back at another time. At the studio I go to, there's a sign at the front of the shop welcoming visitors and inviting them to speak directly to any working artist. You shouldn't be left standing or wandering around for ten minutes without anyone acknowledging your existence. That's poor customer service and doesn't bode well for the treatment you'd get as a client.

THE GRAND TOUR

Before choosing to get a tattoo from any studio, you'll want to talk to the staff and ask them questions about the shop in general. Tell them that you've never been there before and just came by to check the place out. Sometimes they will offer a tour of the facility, but if they don't, politely ask for one. It usually takes only a few minutes, and it can tell you a lot about the shop's customer relations and cleanliness.

You should be shown at least a couple of the workstations, the restroom, and the sterilization room. The workstations should be neat and clean and not have piles of dusty items cluttering up the shelves. There should be a relatively comfortable chair or table for the client, and the chairs should be metal, plastic, or vinyl—because these materials can be sanitized. Some artists will cover their chairs in some kind of plastic barrier that's replaced between clients; that's fine, too. There shouldn't

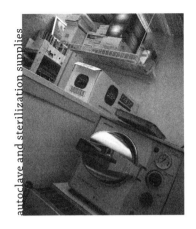

autoclave and sterilization supplies

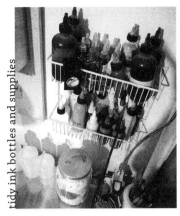

tidy ink bottles and supplies

be any carpeting in the work area; only floors that can be mopped are acceptable. If there isn't an artist currently working, all equipment should be stored away—you shouldn't see any tattoo machines, tubes, needles, or open ink bottles left unattended (unless the artist is just on a short break in the middle of a tattoo).

If there's an artist actively working on a client, watch them for a while if you can. Are they wearing gloves? If they touch anything besides the client (like the phone), they should change gloves. They shouldn't use any spray bottles directly on the client's skin—some use bottles with a pour spout and some spray onto a paper towel and then wipe the client's skin; both are acceptable. Dirty paper towels and gloves should be discarded in a red trash bag marked for biohazardous waste. New needles and tubes should be pulled from a fresh sterilizer pouch. An overall attention to detail and a friendly rapport with the client are both signs of a professional artist.

Even the restroom can give you a good indication of how clean the rest of the shop is. If they can't manage to keep a toilet and sink clean, I'd be very worried about their willingness to take the time to properly sterilize and sanitize their equipment and stations.

The sterilization room, however, is your true destination. Some shops may not have an entire room dedicated to sterilization, which is

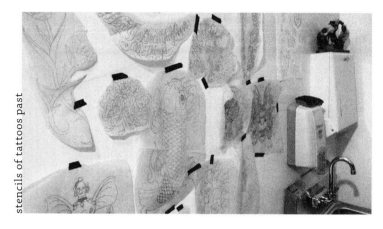

okay, as long as it's an area that's sectioned off and kept clean. If your "tour guide" doesn't point out their autoclave sterilizer, ask about it. You're likely to see an ultrasonic cleaner, a sink for scrubbing tubes and needle bars, sterilizer pouches for use in the autoclave, and maybe even stacks of sterilized items that haven't yet been distributed to the artists. Do all of these things look clean and well organized? Piles of dirty tubes and needle bars, spills on the counters or floor, and a dirty sink are all warning signs. This area should be kept impeccable at all times.

The last thing you want to ask before leaving this room is about the shop's latest spore-test results. Spores are live cells that can reproduce, and if those cells contain dangerous blood-borne diseases or bacteria, they must be eradicated. That is the function of the autoclave sterilizer. But putting the equipment in the sterilizer does little good if the autoclave isn't functioning properly. In order to kill these cells, an autoclave sterilizer has to run at a minimum of 246 degrees Fahrenheit for thirty minutes. Once a month (or two at the most), every autoclave should be tested to ensure it is running at full capacity and killing all spores. That's where the spore strip test comes in. The spore sample is run through the autoclave and then sent to a lab, where it is examined to be sure all the spores are dead. You should ask for the date and results of the last spore strip test conducted on

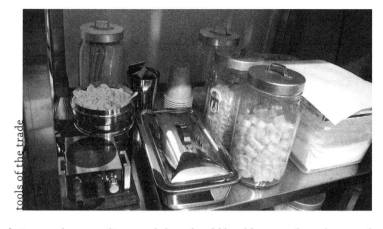

their autoclave sterilizer, and they should be able to produce the actual paperwork for you as proof.

Although the above questions may seem invasive or rude, you have every right to the information, and the shop's employees should have no objection to answering your questions or allowing you to inspect the shop, as long as you are polite and respectful. If they refuse or act insulted by your questions, that's a big red flag that they're hiding something. If the shop is crowded and busy, and you feel it may truly be bad timing, show up again at a slower time (unannounced) and try again. If you sense any bad vibes or see any of the above-mentioned warning signs, it may be prudent to search out a different shop. Never put your life in the hands of someone you don't trust 100 percent.

> *TIP: Some shops you enter may have loud, obnoxious music playing or signs that freely use harsh profanity and insulting language. It's up to you whether you personally find that offensive or not, but I'm not going to patronize a place that doesn't feel the need to make me feel welcome.*

choosing and creating your design

Choosing your tattoo design is a very personal decision, and no one (not even me) can tell you what to get. Sometimes we need a little push in the right direction, though—some inspiration that helps us find that perfect design. That's what this section is for.

When you enter a tattoo shop, you'll no doubt see the flash I mentioned in Chapter 10—pages upon pages of predrawn tattoo designs. A lot of people choose their tattoos directly from these flash sheets, and that's okay if that's what you really want. But you need to realize that those same flash sheets are distributed to hundreds of tattoo shops across the globe, and hundreds of people have likely chosen the exact same tattoo. Since the number one reason for getting inked in the first place is self-expression, it kind of defeats that purpose if you don't use any imagination when choosing your design.

That doesn't mean flash sheets don't serve a valuable purpose. They can be a great starting point for building your perfect tattoo. Use the flash design as inspiration, but change it up—add to it, subtract from it, change

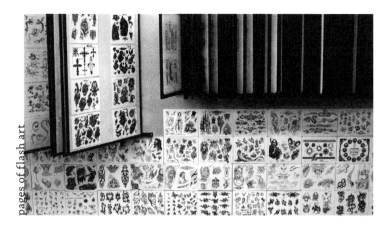
pages of flash art

the colors, change the shape. Do something to make the original drawing more unique. Or you could go completely custom and come up with your very own design. But sometimes that's easier said than done—how do you design a great tattoo from scratch?

✺ Know Its Purpose

What is your reason for wanting a tattoo in the first place? Do you just want one for the sake of having one? Or do you have some special purpose for wanting it? People get tattoos for many reasons, and as long as you have accepted the fact that it will be permanent, then there are no wrong reasons.

If you just want a tattoo because they're pretty, then think about what things you find pretty. Flowers, birds, butterflies, trees, hearts—there are many options that satisfy the need for something feminine. When people ask me why I chose to get fairies, flowers, strawberries, and butterflies, my answer is simple: Those things make me happy. And I like being able to look at my artwork every day and have it bring a smile to my face. If you find something pretty that makes you smile, it just might make a good tattoo choice for you.

If you have a deeper reason for wanting a tattoo, then think about that reason and what it means to you. Wanting a tattoo that truly reflects who you are as a person can be the most difficult concept to translate into a picture, but it's not impossible. Think about the things that are most important to you. Search books, magazines, the Internet, and any other resources you can find that focus on those things you love. If you take the time to really search—within yourself as well— you'll find something that speaks to you. Don't give up until you find exactly what you're looking for. It may be one small thing, or you could decide to put several elements together. And don't sell yourself short on what you really want because you're afraid it will be too expensive or too painful!

If you want to get a tattoo in honor of someone else, you have to think a little differently. Whether they are still alive or have passed on, this tattoo should reflect what they love or find important. If your grandmother is always baking cookies, then a cookie might be a perfectly appropriate tattoo in her honor. If your uncle was a fisherman, then a fish or fishing equipment might be the right design. Even your mother's favorite piece of jewelry can be turned into a tattoo. When you choose a qualified and talented artist, your options are almost limitless.

∽ Details

There are some limits to what an artist can do with your design idea. Some things simply have too much detail to look good if you're willing to have only a four-inch tattoo. Small tattoos just can't accommodate a lot of detail; over time, as the lines spread out, they can blend together and look like one dark blob. If you want detail, you have to be willing to get a larger tattoo.

The only major exception to that rule I know of is artist Anil Gupta. He owns Inkline Studio in New York City and is noted for his miniature masterpieces. He has replicated numerous famous paintings, such as the *Mona Lisa* and *The Birth of Venus*, in a size just slightly larger than a quarter. His work is so fine and detailed that I believe it will stand the test of time.

☙ Colors

The color of your skin and the color(s) of the design you're wanting need to be taken into consideration as well. If you're a very dark-skinned person, your artist may advise against a tattoo with light colors that won't show up well. You may need to stick to darker, bolder colors that will stand the test of time.

No matter what color your skin is, the color(s) of your tattoo need to be thought out in advance, especially if you have sensitive skin, are prone to allergic reactions, or spend a lot of time in the sun.

If you have sensitive skin or are prone to allergic reactions, you might want to avoid getting the color red in your tattoo. No matter what the brand of ink or how safe the ingredients, some people have reactions to the materials used to make red pigments. If you really want red in your tattoo but are concerned about a possible reaction, you can arrange to have your artist do a test patch in an inconspicuous area. But keep in mind that a test patch doesn't come with free removal—if you do have a reaction, you, not your artist, are responsible for the consequences.

If you spend a lot of time in the sun, bright colors fade fastest. Even if you use sunscreen all the time, your tattoo will eventually show wear from sun exposure and tanning. Yellows, oranges, and reds fade the fastest; greens and blues hold for a while; and black is your most stable color option. You can still get bright colors if you want them, but be prepared to need a touch-up every couple of years to keep it looking good.

☙ Creating the Tattoo

Once you have an idea in your head, turning it into a tattoo is not as daunting as it might seem. You don't have much drawing talent? That's what your tattoo artist is for. Your job is to bring as many references to your artist as possible and to be able to describe your vision with as much detail as possible.

Photo references can come from anywhere—books, magazines, actual photographs, movie covers, posters, advertisements, candy wrappers—

whatever shows some kind of depiction of what you're looking for. Bring in several references that show different aspects of your idea if you need to. For example, let's say you want a tattoo of a frog sitting on a lily pad next to a lotus flower. You could bring in two or three pictures of frogs you like—maybe you like one for the pose, one for the colors, and another for the shape of its feet. And you could also bring in several lotus flower and lily pad references for different aspects you like of each one, and ask your artist to put them all together into the one picture you have in your mind.

If you can or want to draw out your idea, go for it. But don't be offended if your artist redraws it for the actual tattoo. They know how designs need to work to create the best tattoo, and that's not always the same as it may be on paper. They will also take into consideration the part of your body where the tattoo will be placed and how the design will best flow with your shape in that area.

❧ Artist's Fees

If you want your artist to draw or design something large or complicated, they may charge an artist's fee. That fee protects the artist from wasting their time by drawing up a design and then having you decide you don't want the tattoo, or taking it to someone else to get it done. The fee should be reasonable, and it should be applied to the cost of the tattoo when you get it. Make sure you get that in writing so there is no confusion later.

> *TIP: Here's a little insider secret for you—most tattoo artists love custom work. They get tired of doing the same old flash day in and day out, and the opportunity to be creative is a real treat for them. Give them a little artistic freedom, and they may even cut you a deal on the price. But even if they don't, most artists put their heart and soul into a custom piece, and the extra effort really shows in the end. You get the most bang for your buck when you allow your artist to do what he/she does best.*

choosing
your artist

If choosing and getting a tattoo is a big decision, then choosing the person you're going to trust to mark you indelibly is even more of one! Before you decide who to hand your hard-earned money and body to, here are some things you'll want to consider first.

๛ Cleanliness

The big "C-word" again. Getting a beautiful tattoo won't seem so great if you also contract a disease or get an infection. It's very important to be sure that your artist is working in a clean and sterile studio and follows Standard Precautions themselves. If studios must be licensed in your state, then make sure it is. If artists must be certified, make sure he/she is. Usually a clean studio means a clean artist, but don't take that for granted. Watch them work on other clients and ask them questions about their sterilization procedures.

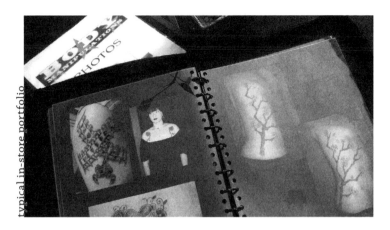

typical in-store portfolio

TIP: True professionals will not be offended by questions and will be happy to answer them, but they may not want to do so while working on a client. So don't feel affronted if they want to talk with you at another time. Some artists prefer not to be distracted when they are working, which is a good thing if you're the one sitting in their chair!

✍ Talent and Experience

A clean and safe tattoo does not necessarily make a beautiful tattoo. So after you've determined that a tattooer is safe, you'll want to see how good they are as an artist.

Most artists will have a portfolio available at the shop or on the Internet. It's easy to get swept up in looking through a portfolio—you see bright colors and cool designs, and can easily be fooled into thinking the artistry is good, too. When examining a portfolio, you need to slow down and really look at it with a critical eye. Remember, this is someone you're considering hiring to mark you for life!

When looking at the portfolio, pay attention to details. A lot of tattooers can do a cute-looking fairy at first glance, but take a close look at the face, hands, or feet—that's where a lot of inexperienced artists mess up. Body parts shouldn't have dark, harsh lines outlining them unless it's a cartoon character. Circles should look like circles, and all lines should be smooth and continuous, not choppy or shaky. Shading should also be smooth, and you shouldn't see a definite line where the shading begins or ends. Coloring should be even and solid, not dark in some places and faded in others.

Consistency is also very important. As you look through the portfolio, does the level of quality look consistent from one picture to another, or do some of them look much better or worse than others? You never know what kind of day you'll catch an inconsistent artist on, and you don't want to be sitting in the chair on a bad one.

> *TIP: Keep in mind that photos in portfolios can be stolen and copied from other artists. If it looks like a signature or copyright frame has been removed from the photos, or if you have any reason to question the authenticity of the portfolio art, be very wary of that tattooer. It doesn't happen often, but it does happen, especially on the Internet.*

✍ Expertise

You may think that "expertise" is just another word for "talent," but not in this case. I'm speaking of genre expertise here. Just because an artist is talented and experienced does not mean he/she would be the best choice for the particular design you are wanting.

For example, Paul Booth of Last Rites Tattoo Theatre is one of the most famous tattoo artists in the business. His waiting list of clients is around two years, and people are happy to wait that long just to get inked by him. He is amazingly talented, but his specialty—his expertise—is black-and-gray biomechanical and horror art. Asking Paul Booth to do a dainty little butterfly would be ridiculous.

Every artist has either a specialty or a genre they prefer to work in. Find an artist who has expertise in the style of tattoo you're looking for. That doesn't mean you have to find an artist who specializes in

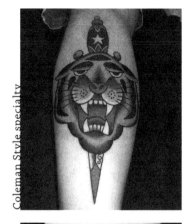

Coleman Style specialty

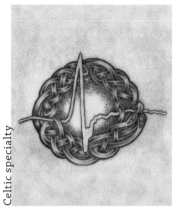

Celtic specialty

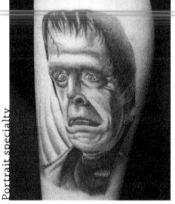

Portrait specialty

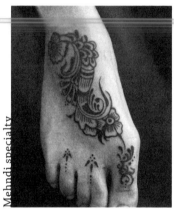

Mehndi specialty

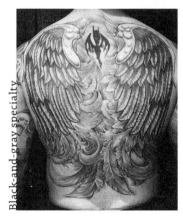

Black-and-gray specialty

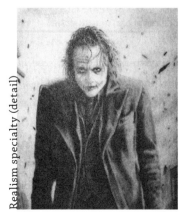

Realism specialty (detail)

strawberries if that's what you want, but if you want your strawberries to be realistic, then you want an artist who specializes in realism. If you want your strawberries to be bold and colorful, then you want an artist who really understands color, not one who prefers to work only with black ink. If you want a portrait, you definitely want an artist who can pull off a great portrait.

The artists themselves will help you in this part of your search. Some of them will tell you right up front that they don't specialize in the kind of tattoo you're wanting. Or you'll get the sense that they're really not excited about the idea you are presenting to them. If they don't want to do it, forcing them will only make both of you unhappy. Artists who really like an idea will do their best at it, making you a happy customer.

৩ Congeniality

Although you may know them for only a few hours your entire life, a friendly artist whom you can personally connect with is important.

Sometimes different personalities just don't mesh, and you don't want to enter into a business relationship with someone you can't relate to, or vice versa. You do have to talk with them and will basically be at their mercy once they start working on you—it does help if they actually like you.

If the tattoo you're getting is large, and you may be spending several hours—or even several sessions—in close proximity to your artist, it's even more important to have good chemistry.

price and tipping

"Good tattoos ain't cheap, and cheap tattoos ain't good."

—UNKNOWN

The old adage may not be eloquent, but its undeniable accuracy has made it one of the most popular slogans in the tattoo industry.

That isn't to say that an expensive tattoo automatically makes a good tattoo, but unless you are good friends with a really good artist, you're not going to get a great tattoo for dirt cheap—and a great tattoo is the ultimate goal here, right?

How Much Does a Tattoo Actually Cost?

Every artist charges a different rate for work, and prices vary depending on size, detail, and colors. The average range is anywhere between $50 and $250 per hour. That's a pretty big range, because a lot of variables go into determining how much an artist can charge for time.

Shop Minimum

Most shops have an absolute minimum they have to charge for each tattoo in order to cover their overhead. Even the tiniest tattoo still requires artists to pull out all their equipment and then clean and sterilize everything afterward. That minimum fee is your insurance policy for a clean and safe tattoo and runs between $50 and $75.

Overhead

Some shops have higher overheads than others, and therefore have to charge more for their tattoos to keep up with the bills. Some state and city laws require tattoo studios to carry expensive licensing, certification, or insurance policies that neighboring shops may not be required to have.

Location

Local economy affects how much a tattoo artist can charge and still stay in business. Shops in smaller towns with a lower economy won't be able to charge as much as big, booming city shops. Even real estate location within a town can create a price difference between one shop and another; if one is much more conveniently located or in a busier section of town, it may charge more.

Competition

The amount of competition in a particular town can have a great impact on tattoo prices. The more competition, or the better the competition, the more a shop is forced to lower prices.

Demand

If a shop happens to be very popular or is home to a world-renowned artist, prices are bound to go up. Artists who are in high demand can set their rates as high as they want, as long as their clients are willing to pay.

∽ Don't Haggle

If you're a bargain hunter who loves to clip coupons and haggle at yard sales, this is neither the time nor the place. Once an artist has set a price, your options are to either take it or leave it. Haggling is disrespectful and won't do you any good anyway.

If you know from the outset that you are on a budget, let them know that up front. Tell them what your limit is and ask them if they can work your design within that limit. If not, you may simply need to wait until you have saved enough money to get what you want.

∽ How Much Are You Worth?

It amazes me how some people won't bat an eye at throwing down a couple hundred dollars on a new outfit or cell phone—which will be obsolete or tossed away within a year—but then complain about having to spend the same money on something that will be with them for the rest of their life. Even if you're not one to usually spend a lot on yourself, be prepared to splurge when you get a tattoo.

When considering how much you want to spend on a tattoo, you should also consider how much you value yourself. Your tattoo will become a part of you—literally. It makes a statement to others about who you are. What will your tattoo say about you?

∽ Tipping

Tipping your tattoo artist is not required, but it is a nice gesture. When you're already shelling out a couple hundred dollars on a tattoo, you may think it's a bit rich of the artist to want a tip on top of it. But oftentimes, the artist gets only a percentage of the actual tattoo fee. Most of it goes to the shop owner, who pays for the artists' supplies and gives them a place to work. Most tattoo artists are struggling day to day just like the rest of us and can really use a little extra cash. Plus, it's nice just to show appreciation for their hard work.

So, how much is right? Some people tip just as they would at a restaurant—10 percent for good service, 15 percent for great service, and 20 percent for excellent, above-and-beyond service. But there's really no hard and fast rule. Even if you can spare only an extra five or ten bucks, it's going to be greatly appreciated. A lot of customers don't tip at all, but that doesn't mean you shouldn't either.

If you didn't have any cash or just forgot to tip, go back the next day or even the next week if you have to. It's never too late to say thank you.

TIP: An artist's tip doesn't always have to come in the form of cash. A batch of homemade muffins or cookies is sometimes even more exciting than money! One time, I delivered an entire home-cooked meal to my artist and her crew. These guys work long hours and don't get good food very often. It's a great, unique way to show your appreciation.

setting and keeping the appointment

Once you've decided on your design and your artist, and you've saved up enough money, it's time to get that tattoo! The first thing you'll need to do is set an appointment. But there's more involved in doing that than you'd think.

First off, getting a tattoo is not a process you want to rush. Even a small tattoo should not be scheduled on a lunch break or on a day when you have a million other things to do. Make sure you pick a day when you can relax during and after the procedure.

Another thing to consider are those self-imposed restrictions I mentioned earlier. For the first couple of weeks, you'll need to baby your tattoo as it heals. There will be no hot-tubbing, swimming, or soaking in the bathtub. You need to keep your tattoo out of the sun as much as possible, since you won't be able to apply sunscreen to it in the first few weeks. Sweat and dirt or excessive flexing of the muscles in the area of the tattoo can lead to problems. If you have anything coming up in your schedule that would involve any of these things—swim meets, athletic competitions, vacation on the beach—then the tattoo should wait until your schedule opens up again.

∽ Mutual Respect

Once you have officially set your appointment, have the courtesy to show up—on time—or call your artist with as much advance notice as possible that you won't be able to make it. Your artist's time is valuable, and standing them up is a no-no. And if you show up half an hour late, don't expect your artist to be able to squeeze you in. They may have taken a walk-in job or just simply be annoyed enough to not want to deal with you that day.

Even though you should show up on time for your appointment, you may have to wait for your artist to be ready for you. If an earlier client's appointment is taking longer than expected, you don't want the artist to rush that job any more than you'd want them to rush yours. Bring something to entertain yourself with in case this happens and wait patiently. You shouldn't have to wait longer than thirty minutes, though. It would be impolite for the artist to be that far behind and not give you the option to reschedule.

∽ The Brush-Off

Sometimes—although it's rare—an artist will stand up the client. The artist either won't be there at all or will be fully involved in a large piece on another client, with no possibility of finishing anywhere near the time of the appointment you set. This is extremely unprofessional, and if this happens to you, I suggest you find another artist. Tattooers who do this are generally the types who fall into this kind of problem due to bad time management, so they're likely to do the same thing over again. If you've already put down a deposit, you can ask for it back, but your chances of getting it are slim. You can take the tattooer to civil court for the deposit, but honestly, sometimes it's better to just let it go and move on. Find a better artist—there are plenty out there.

food, drink, medication, and drugs

We all know that we need to take care of our bodies for overall health, and this becomes even more important when your body is trying to mend itself. Everything from the food you eat to the prescription drugs you take can alter your state of health and thus your ability to heal.

✌ Proper Nutrition

Eating a balanced diet, low in sugar and fat, and high in fiber and nutrients, is the best way to keep your body's defenses at their peak. But certain vitamins are particularly advantageous to your immune system— vitamins A, C, and E and the minerals zinc and selenium. Taking these vitamins for at least a week before and after your tattoo can do more good toward healing a tattoo than the best aftercare ointment.

Caffeine and refined sugars, however, drain the body of these necessary nutrients and should be avoided as much as possible. You may find that making these alterations to your diet will make you feel better in many other ways, too!

ഏ Alcohol

Do not drink before getting a tattoo. The main reason for this is that alcohol thins the blood and can make you bleed excessively while getting inked. This not only makes it more difficult for your artist to execute a smooth tattoo, but it can also lead to heavy scabbing that could actually damage the tattoo afterward.

Another reason not to drink is that if your artist senses that you have any alcohol in your system, he/she won't tattoo you. You can't legally sign the release form if you're impaired.

ഏ Over-the-Counter Medications and Holistic/Herbal Remedies

Most over-the-counter medications are safe and won't prevent you from getting a tattoo or cause problems. But aspirin or anything else that has a blood-thinning effect can cause bleeding difficulties just like alcohol.

You may be tempted to take a painkiller before getting a tattoo to take the edge off, but that isn't necessary. And taking anything with aspirin in it just before getting inked is definitely not a good idea.

It's unknown just how the body may be affected by herbal supplements or holistic treatments, but there have been rare cases of someone's body rejecting the ink or not healing properly due to the presence of certain herbal supplements.

ഏ Prescription Drugs

Blood thinners are by and large the biggest concern when you're getting inked. Anything that can cause an excess of bleeding will complicate a tattoo. The artist will have a difficult time laying a clean tattoo with all the blood hindering any efforts. The flow of blood could also flush out some of the ink and create faded areas. The resulting scabs could also hinder proper healing of your tattoo. If you're on any kind of blood thinner, do not get a tattoo.

The next big culprit seems to be prescription acne medications—benzoyl peroxide and oral retinoids, such as Accutane, all pose a risk in relation to getting a tattoo. Not a health risk, but a risk to the ink itself.

Benzoyl peroxide is a powerful bleaching agent and can fade tattoos, as well as clothing. New tattoos are the most at risk because the new protective layers of epidermis haven't fully formed. This is another reason why you shouldn't get tattooed in an area where you are prone to acne breakouts. Prescription-strength benzoyl peroxide, if used regularly over a tattoo, can potentially fade it as well.

Accutane has a high incidence of complaints in relation to tattoos. Many patients report increased pain due to heightened skin sensitivity. Other complications are scarring from the tattoo procedure and even rejection of the ink. Accutane patients should allow plenty of time—at least three months—for the drug to work its way out of their system before attempting to get a tattoo, and shouldn't resume treatment until it's healed.

✂ Illegal Drugs

There is a misconception that tattoo artists are of the "rock star" mentality and are cool with the use of illegal drugs. This is not the case with most of them, and even if some do use illegal drugs recreationally on their own time, they have enough sense not to when they're working. Getting and giving tattoos requires a clear head.

Using illegal drugs is obviously not a good idea, but it's especially problematic when you're getting a tattoo. An artist won't work on someone who's intoxicated or otherwise impaired.

what to bring with you

There is one item you absolutely must bring to a tattoo appointment, or you'll be turned away: a valid state ID or driver's license. Without legal proof of age, you cannot be tattooed. The artist and studio owner risk losing their licensing if they tattoo someone without having a copy of the client's ID along with a consent form.

Money, too, is another necessary thing to bring with you. Not all tattoo shops accept credit cards and very few accept checks. But cash is always accepted—and don't forget to bring a little extra for a tip.

Other than your ID and money, anything else you might bring is up to you. But if you're nervous about getting a tattoo, don't like the sound of the tattoo machine, or are going to be there for a while, here are some suggestions of items you may want to have on hand.

❧ A Friend

Okay, so a friend isn't an "item," but you still might want to have one with you. Most artists are okay with your having a friend join you in the work area while getting inked, but always ask first to be sure. A companion can distract you or make you laugh during the more painful parts of the tattoo, or they can simply keep you company if you want someone to talk to.

✑ Something to Read

If your artist isn't the chatty type, or if you just need a distraction, bringing along a book or magazine can help. It will also give you something to do if you have to wait a bit for your appointment.

✑ Music/MP3 Player

Listening to music can soothe you if you're nervous about getting tattooed. It can also block out the sound of the tattoo machine if that's something you don't particularly like.

✑ Gum

Chewing gum can help deal with anxiety before the tattoo and reduce pain during the process.

✑ Something to Drink

Although most artists won't want you snacking in the work area during the tattoo, a drink is usually okay. You've already learned that eating before your tattoo is important to keep up your blood glucose levels, but if you're not able to do that, then at least get some juice or a soda. Plus, you might just get thirsty while sitting through the tattoo.

> *TIP: DO NOT bring young children with you to your appointment. Although I'm definitely a proponent of exposing your kids to the beauty of tattoos, young children don't like to sit through a tattoo session and usually just end up distracting the artists. It's not the shop employees' job to watch your kids while you get a tattoo; if you can't find someone to care for them, reschedule your appointment for a time when you can.*

what to expect

If you've never gotten a tattoo before, sitting in that chair for the first time can be an intimidating experience. If you're nervous, you're not alone. Almost everyone has a sense of anxiety before getting inked for the first time, and sometimes that nervousness persists with each following tattoo.

Knowing what to expect can help ease some of that fear of the unknown. While you're digesting the information in this chapter, keep this one thought tucked away in the back of your head: If getting a tattoo was a terrible experience, people wouldn't go back repeatedly for more ink!

∞ Preparing the Design

The first thing your artist will do—either before or at the beginning of your appointment—is draw up the design. Do not give the drawing your okay until you are 100 percent happy with it. Remember, this is going to be on your body for the rest of your life, and taking an extra ten minutes to change something is worth it. Once you give the drawing the thumbs-up, your artist will create a stencil.

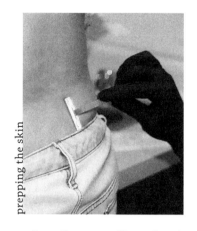

prepping the skin

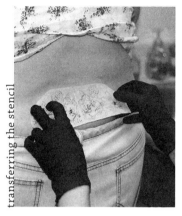

transferring the stencil

Stencils are usually made using a machine called a Thermofax. It's kind of like a copy machine, but it creates a copy by applying heat to a special kind of paper that reacts to the heat to produce the image. Once that is done, your design is ready to be applied to skin.

∽ Prepping the Skin

Your skin needs to be clean and smooth before applying the transfer, so your artist will wipe down your skin (usually with Green Soap) and then—if needed—shave the area. Paper towels should be used for wiping the skin and a disposable razor should be used for shaving—and then both should be discarded in the trash.

Next, your artist may apply a little A+D ointment, K-Y jelly, or deodorant to your skin in order to help the stencil stick. None of these things should come directly in contact with you in their containers—they should be first applied to a paper towel or clean swab and then applied to your skin.

∽ The Stencil Transfer

The stencil is transferred to your body like a temporary tattoo. It's pressed onto the skin, and when the paper is peeled away, you'll have a beautiful purple outline of your design. At this point, you will be given the chance to check it out in the mirror.

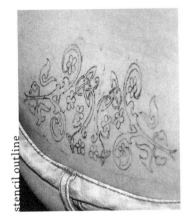
stencil outline

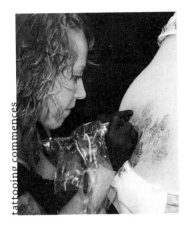
tattooing commences

This is where a lot of people get excited and lose their objectivity. Keep your head, because it's really important to look closely at your stencil in the mirror and make sure it is positioned exactly right. If it needs to be tilted to the right or left, raised or lowered, or even if you suddenly realize a key element is missing, this is the time to say something! It's not a big deal for the artist to erase the stencil and try again. Once they start the actual tattoo, there's no turning back.

✑ The First Strokes of the Needle

If it hasn't been done already, this is when your artist will get out all the equipment to get started on your tattoo.

The first needle, which is used to do the outline of the design, is called a liner. A liner is usually not just a single needle, but a small cluster of sharps in a circular shape. First you'll hear the buzz of the machine and then your artist will rub a little ointment onto your skin, lean toward you, and place the tip against your skin for the first time.

You can stop holding your breath now. . . .

The first line is always the hardest. A lot of people tense up in anticipation of that first pass of the needle, which actually makes it hurt more than it should. After a few strokes, though, you will start to relax and realize that it's not so bad. I can't tell you how many times I've heard

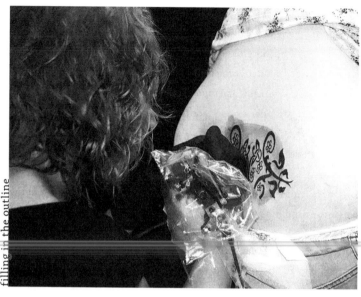
filling in the outline

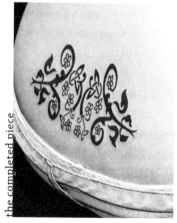
the completed piece

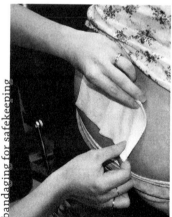
bandaging for safekeeping

the phrase "That wasn't nearly as bad as I expected," after someone got their first tattoo. But no one seems to believe it until they experience it themselves.

Every once in a while, your artist will wipe down your skin with some Green Soap, and you'll be able to get a good look at the progress up to that point.

Once the outlines are all finished, it's time to fill or color in the tattoo. This is where the piece really comes to life. Before beginning this step, though, your artist will change needles and sometimes even change machines. A machine with larger coils provides more power to push a larger needle group. The type of needle group generally used to do shading and fill color is called a magnum, or "mag" for short. Instead of being circular in shape, the sharps are set in a couple of flat rows. This allows the artist to fill a large area more quickly.

Some people claim that coloring is more painful than outlining, but it differs from one person to another. The good thing about coloring is that it's done in shorter spurts, whereas long lines have to be done in one solid stroke with no breaks.

> *TIP: Don't avoid color just to avoid pain! Some people will decide that they don't want any shading or coloring in their tattoo because they're afraid it's going to hurt more. Shading and color are what really add personality to a design, and it's all going to hurt a little bit, so just go for it. It'll be over before you know it, and the end results make it worth any discomfort.*

taking a break

If your tattoo is small enough, you may not require any breaks during the session. To be honest, breaks are inconvenient—both to you and to the artist—but everyone needs them sometimes.

Tattoos that take a couple of hours or more are likely to get interrupted by either the artist or the client needing a break—whether that be a bathroom break, a smoke break, or simply to be able to get up and stretch.

Too many breaks can irritate the other party—the artist may get annoyed if the client needs them to stop too often, and the client obviously doesn't appreciate having the artist disrespecting their time when they are paying for it. Even if you're in pain, taking multiple breaks will only make it worse. It's best to just stick through it as long as you can.

If you do take a break to go outside, especially if you're going to smoke, your artist should put a temporary bandage over your tattoo in order to protect it from bacteria and airborne toxins.

split sessions

If the tattoo you're getting is very large, and you're not able to sit through the entire tattoo in one visit—due to either money, time, or discomfort— you can split it up into multiple sessions. No session should be less than two hours, though; if you really can't even sit through that much, you might consider getting a smaller tattoo.

∾ Money

Getting a tattoo, especially a large one, can be quite expensive. If you don't have all the money for the entire piece at once, you can ask your artist to split it up into bits you can afford (within reason). I recently had my artist do a large piece on my arm, and each time I went in for a session, I told her how much I could spend that day, which determined how much work she would do on it that day. Obviously, this kind of arrangement has to be made before starting the tattoo—you can't tell the artist afterward that you don't have enough money!

✑ Time

If you don't have enough time to sit through a long tattoo, you can ask your artist about splitting it up into shorter sessions that fit into your schedule better. This should also be arranged ahead of time, out of respect for your artist, so they know not to block out their availability for the whole piece.

✑ Discomfort

If you've never gotten a tattoo before, you probably don't know how much time under the needle you can tolerate. If you have, though, and you know you can handle only two, three, or four hours at a time, there's no reason to push yourself beyond what you can reasonably take. Even if you have agreed to a three-hour session and you're having difficulty with the pain after two and a half hours, it's okay to ask your artist to stop a little early. Not if the tattoo is almost finished, though! This is only for larger pieces that have enough left to necessitate another session.

✑ Finishing Up

When all the shading and coloring is finished, your artist will give your tattoo a good wipe-down and let you take a look. Again, really look at it and make sure you don't see anything missing or incorrect. If it's to your liking, your artist will rub some more ointment on you and bandage you up. Congratulations! You are now the proud owner of a piece of living art.

✑ Before You Leave

After your tattoo is completed, you'll need to pay for your new ink. Remember to tip if you can. You should also be given aftercare instructions. Some studios even give you the supplies you need to care for your tattoo for the next week, or at least sell the products they recommend. But just in case they don't, or if you're in doubt about the instructions they do give you, the next section covers what you need to know about caring for your new tattoo.

aftercare and the healing process

From the moment you leave the tattoo shop with your new ink, it becomes your responsibility to keep it clean and safe from germs and irritants. If you were given instructions about what to do by your artist, follow those before you follow mine. If you trusted your artist enough to give you the tattoo, then you should trust them enough to advise you on how to care for it.

However, we all like a second opinion sometimes, and when it comes to caring for a tattoo, there are a lot of opinions. Even among professional artists, there are dozens of differing opinions on what works best. If you ask ten artists what product they recommend for tattoo aftercare, you're likely to get ten different answers.

Unraveling the Aftercare Mystery

Why are there so many different products and recommendations? Well, because people are different and everyone likes different things. The fact is, most tattoos would heal on their own even if you didn't do anything special to them at all except wash them. Ointments and other aftercare products only help make the healing process more comfortable or a little shorter.

So, the two basic rules of healing a tattoo are: (1) keep it clean, and (2) keep it moist. What you choose to use to accomplish these two things is pretty much up to you. Take into consideration what you like and what your skin responds best to. There are only a few products most artists will agree that you should not use, although there have been no clinical studies to prove the claims of adverse effects.

PETROLEUM JELLY

This product was the most widely used and recommended aftercare product back in the early days of tattooing. But since then, people have discovered that petroleum jelly isn't the best thing for tattoos. A lot of people claim that it actually draws the new ink away from the skin and can lead to a faded tattoo. It's also been suggested that petroleum jelly clogs pores and can lead to infection.

But what about aftercare products that contain petrolatum? Although some people advise against it, I personally recommend some aftercare products that list petrolatum among the ingredients, as long as it's not the primary ingredient. Using a product that has a little bit, though, is fine and perfectly safe for most users.

HYDROGEN PEROXIDE

Many of us grew up with moms who insisted that every wound be treated with hydrogen peroxide for its bacteria-fighting properties. It turns out, though, that it really isn't very effective in warding off bacteria. What it does ward off are white blood cells and fibroblasts (cells that repair wounds), making it more difficult for your skin to heal itself. So maybe Mom wasn't always right.

NEOSPORIN (ALSO KNOWN AS TRIPLE ANTIBIOTIC)

Neosporin was once used and highly recommended to heal all wounds, including tattoos, but it's been found to cause an allergic reaction for a lot of people. A reaction to Neosporin produces dozens of tiny red bumps that can scar and ruin your tattoo.

"BAD" INGREDIENTS (ESPECIALLY FOR SENSITIVE SKIN)

Anything that contains the following could cause an adverse reaction: lanolin, beeswax, menthol, dyes, and perfumes. There is no way for me (or your artist) to know how your body might react to any of these things, so watch out for these ingredients and try to stay away from products that have them.

> *TIP: Lanolin hypersensitivity is a very common problem, yet many companies still use it in their products. Lanolin is a fatty substance that comes from the sebaceous glands of sheep. Lanolin has waterproofing properties that protect sheep's wool from getting soaked in the rain. Lanolin is extracted from the wool and used in many lotions, ointments, and cosmetics. If you break out in itchy rashes you can't explain, you may want to check the ingredients of some of your cosmetics and lotions.*

Now, on to discussing what you *can* use!

Keeping Your Tattoo Clean

Since the number one goal is to keep your tattoo clean at all times, you're going to have to wash it—usually at least twice a day. Harsh or abrasive soaps can irritate your tattoo or cause an adverse reaction, so it's important that you use something mild that doesn't contain chemicals. Liquid or foam soaps are always preferable to bar soaps because you reduce the risk of cross-contamination.

Again, at this point, the decision is yours as long as you stick to the basic rules, but here are a few suggestions in case you are at a loss.

SATIN THERAPEUTIC SKIN CLEANSER

This is my all-time favorite and top choice. Satin is an antimicrobial cleanser, rather than antibacterial. It's much milder but more effective against various microorganisms than antibacterial soap. It's got a bit of a sterile scent to it, which some don't care for, but it's really a great product—I use it for washing my face, too. Satin is sold at a lot of tattoo studios, and it's available through some online companies.

PROVON ANTIMICROBIAL SOAP

Provon is just as good as Satin, but seems to be a little harder to find. Made by the same company as Purell hand sanitizer, Provon soap comes in a foam or liquid antimicrobial wash. Provon can sometimes be found at tattoo studios. You can also ask your pharmacist if they keep any behind the counter; you won't need a prescription, but it can be hard to find on regular store shelves. If they don't carry the specific brand, they may have something comparable.

ANTIBACTERIAL SOAP

If you can't find an antimicrobial cleanser, then an antibacterial soap will suffice. I recommend buying off-brand, though, because generics tend to be milder and not so harsh on the skin.

PURE OR NATURAL CLEANSERS

If you're more organically inclined, natural cleansers are fine as long as they don't contain any of the "bad" ingredients listed previously. Pure soaps, however, like castile soap, can tend to be a bit harsh for some people—especially if they contain peppermint or eucalyptus oils. So be careful and discontinue using anything if it starts giving you problems.

✎ Aftercare Options

After you have washed your tattoo, you'll need to apply some kind of ointment or lotion product to aid the healing process and keep your skin soft. This is where an actual aftercare product may come into play—and where the real confusion begins.

The main purpose of an aftercare product is to keep the tattoo moist. Keeping your tattoo from drying out is important because it can crack, bleed, and be quite painful if it's allowed to get too dry. Just the natural movements of the body will flex and stretch your tattoo to its limits sometimes, but keeping it supple will allow it to accommodate those movements.

It's good to have an ointment that has a bacteria-fighting agent to ward off infection, but it's not absolutely necessary. If you're keeping the tattoo clean and wash it immediately after any potentially dangerous exposure, there is little need for it. Your body will heal itself over time, which brings us back to the main purpose of aftercare ointment—moisture.

KISS: Keep It Simple, Stupid

I am a major proponent of sticking with the basics. I haven't always been that way. I've bought into many products that were supposed to make my life easier and provide superior quality over old-fashioned means and methods. You know what I've learned from all that stuff? That there's still nothing that cleans better than good ole baking soda and vinegar, and it doesn't cost an arm and a leg for a fancy bottle. I keep this simplistic view when it comes to aftercare, too.

Yes, you can choose from a wide range of pricey products specifically designed to heal a tattoo—from Tattoo Goo to H2Ocean, there's a long list of companies now making lubes, lotions, and oils that all claim to be the best for caring for your new ink. And of course people will endorse the products when they try them, because they all work! They all work because they all provide one basic service—they keep your tattoo moist. But so does the following list of easy-to-find and inexpensive products.

A+D OINTMENT

I'll admit that there is a major contradiction here because regular A+D ointment contains three of the ingredients you're supposed to avoid:

petrolatum, lanolin, and fragrance. So why do I recommend it? Because it works. It has been and still remains my preferred aftercare product for all of my tattoos, and it's highly recommended by many artists. I have never had an issue with it, but as every person is different, there will still be those who have problems with it. If you decide to try it and experience any issues, stop using it. I will note that A+D has a distinct odor to it that many people find unappealing.

If you have access to it, medical-grade A+D ointment is better than the yellow, brown, and white tube designed for diaper rash, but I use the original ointment with no adverse effects.

AQUAPHOR

This is another product that contains taboo ingredients—petrolatum and lanolin—and yet it's been touted as one of the best aftercare products available. I haven't used this product for healing a tattoo, but I do use it for dry skin and it's fantastic. Hydrophor is a very similar product by a different name and is just as effective.

VITAMIN E

Vitamin E oil or cream will keep the skin supple through the healing stages and is just as effective as any of the products listed so far. And if you happen to have sensitivity issues with petroleum or lanolin, vitamin E doesn't contain those ingredients.

EUCERIN

This product also contains lanolin alcohol, but it's one of the last ingredients in the list. It is known to be a very good all-around lotion. This is what I use after using A+D for the first three or four days. Some artists will tell you to just use lotion from day one, and that's fine as long as you don't have a problem with it. I don't like the feeling of lotion on a sore tattoo, so I prefer a soothing ointment for the first few days.

LUBRIDERM

This is a highly recommended lotion, although I found that it made my tattooed skin burn when I applied it. If you use Lubriderm, make sure you get the dye- and fragrance-free version.

> *NOTE: A relatively new product that has recently been touted as an effective aftercare means is pure emu oil. It's derived from the meat of the flightless bird, which is then filtered and processed until an almost completely pure product is produced. While it is neither inexpensive nor easy to find, I have tried it and have had great success with it. It softens the skin, protects the tattoo, and, since it contains absolutely no other ingredients, is safe for almost everyone to use. Granted, emu oil is not vegan friendly, so it's up to individuals to decide how they feel about using this type of product.*

Too Much of a Good Thing

No matter what product you use to treat your tattoo, the biggest mistake most people make is using too much. Even a great product can produce bad results if you spread it on too thick over a healing tattoo.

Too much ointment, especially if it contains petrolatum, can flush out your new ink, clog pores, and even lead to infection. This is why petroleum-based products are so mistrusted now. But using the right amount—which is actually very little—shouldn't cause any problems.

Keeping your tattoo moist does not mean keeping it wet; it means not letting it dry out. Whatever you decide to apply to your ink after washing it, this is the general rule of thumb: Apply just barely enough to make it slightly glossy, rub it in really good, and then dab it with a clean cloth to remove any excess. Do this each time you wash your tattoo; applying more ointment throughout the day is not necessary.

✍ Aftercare Instructions

Now that you know the basic rules and how to choose a product that is right for you, here is a breakdown of the steps I recommend and follow myself.

FIRST TWELVE TO FIFTEEN HOURS

Take the bandage off after about an hour or two, and that's it. For at least the first twelve hours, do nothing at all to your tattoo, unless you want to apply some Bactine (see tip below). Don't wash it, don't rebandage it; just leave it alone. Give it time to calm down a bit.

> **NO:** Bathing (quick showers are fine—just no soaking or scrubbing!), swimming, hot-tubbing, tanning, shaving, chemical depilatories (hair removal creams), athletic competitions, or working out.

> *TIP: If there is such a thing as a miracle product, I think Bactine spray would be it. For those first twelve to fifteen hours, while you're basically leaving your new tattoo alone, it's going to burn and sting pretty good; a few spritzes of Bactine spray relieve that burn like nothing else. And, since it also kills germs, you're protecting your tattoo at the same time. This is an unorthodox method that a lot of artists don't recommend, but I think it's pure gold. My artist told me about it, and I've been passing it on ever since. My tattoos still heal beautifully using this product.*

DAYS ONE THROUGH THREE

Wash your tattoo* at least twice a day (more only if you actually get dirty or sweaty) and pat dry with a clean towel. Apply a tiny (tiny!) amount of your ointment of choice, rub it in, and then dab it with a clean cloth to remove excess.

NO: Bathing (again, showers are okay), swimming, hot-tubbing, tanning, shaving, or chemical hair removal creams.

LIMIT: Athletic competitions or working out.

*How you wash your tattoo, especially on the first day, is extremely important. You may notice a clear liquid either seeping from or collected and dried on the surface of your tattoo. Even if you don't see it, you'll probably feel it when you start to wash your tattoo. It will feel slippery and slimy. That clear liquid is called plasma, and it's perfectly normal for your skin to ooze a bit of plasma after getting a tattoo. But if you don't get rid of it in that first day, it will harden and turn to scabs, which are quite uncomfortable and can slow down your healing pace.

The first couple of times you wash your tattoo, use lukewarm water (not hot), your cleanser of choice, and your hand. Wash gently over and over again, applying more soap if needed, until that slippery feeling is completely gone. Then pat it dry and apply your ointment. Continue this practice each time you wash your tattoo until you no longer feel the presence of any plasma.

DAYS FOUR THROUGH TWELVE

Wash your tattoo at least twice a day and then apply your lotion of choice. It is okay to apply lotion over scabs or flaking skin. It's all part of the healing process, and the moisture in the lotion helps to get you through this stage.

NO: Bathing (showers okay, see note), swimming, hot-tubbing, tanning, or chemical hair removal creams. Shaving is acceptable once the skin is smooth with no flakes or scabs.

NOTE ON SHOWERING: Especially after the first few days, you may develop a few scabs over your new tattoo. They won't hurt it as long as they don't come off before they're ready. Hot showers soften scabs and make them very easy to pull off prematurely by scrubbing, towel drying, or applying lotion. Be very careful until the scab rehardens, and wait until it's dry to apply lotion.

❦ The Healing Process

As your tattoo heals over the next seven to fourteen days, it will go through a series of changes. Not everyone experiences exactly the same results, but most do follow a similar pattern.

DAY ONE

The day of your tattoo, you'll be a little sore, and your tattoo may bleed a bit. Bleeding should stop within two hours of your leaving the studio. If it doesn't, you should call your tattoo artist.

Otherwise, your skin may be red around the tattoo and feel a little sore and warm to the touch, but it's not too bad.

DAY TWO

When you wake up the next morning, you may find that your tattoo is tight and the skin is hard to flex. It may also hurt even more than it did the previous day. Washing it and applying ointment will help to soothe it. It's okay if it's still warm to the touch, but the redness should be gone.

DAY THREE

The tight feeling still exists and large pieces may still be slightly warm to the touch, but the pain should be less. At this point, your tattoo feels like a mild sunburn. The skin above the tattoo has died and will turn a whitish color, which makes your tattoo color look dull and faded. This is temporary; your color will brighten back up in a few days.

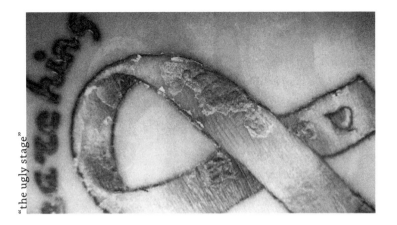
"the ugly stage"

TIP: All tattoos go through what I affectionately call "the ugly stage." This part of the healing process scares a lot of newbies because their once beautiful tattoos now look hideous and ruined. This is all normal, and in just a few more days, the tattoo will regain its original beauty.

DAYS FOUR THROUGH SEVEN

Depending on the size of your tattoo and how quickly your body heals, your tattoo will show the greatest amount of healing during this time. The pain will be minimal. It shouldn't feel warm to the touch, and it may begin to peel and flake. Flakes of skin that have bits of ink in them are perfectly normal. Applying a little extra lotion to drying, flaking skin can help.

The peeling stage is difficult to allow to pass without interference, but *do not* pick or scratch at the flakes. Allow them to fall off on their own. Peeling may lead to bleeding and color loss. The same rule applies to any scabs you may have. They'll fall off when they're ready!

As the dead-skin flakes exfoliate, you'll start noticing the color of your tattoo returning to its original brightness. You'll really notice the difference after each cleaning and lotion application.

DAYS EIGHT THROUGH FOURTEEN

Once the old, dead skin has flaked away, your body has to rebuild new layers of skin to protect your tattoo. It may feel healed at this point, but it's actually a very critical period, and you must continue to protect your ink. You'll need to apply sunscreen any time you'll be out in the sun, even for a short period of time. Your tattoo doesn't have any of the natural defenses the rest of your skin has.

Even after your tattoo is a couple of weeks old and you feel back to normal, you're still only partway there. It takes about three months for your skin to completely regain its structure, so your tattoo is still considered vulnerable until then. Because of that, avoid tanning and the application of any chemical depilatories (hair removal).

Once your tattoo has reached that three-month point, it has officially become a part of you. But that doesn't mean you don't have to continue taking care of it. Keeping your tattoo looking bright and beautiful requires a lifetime of care.

> *TIP: While your tattoo is healing, there will be times when it will itch like crazy. It's so tempting to scratch, but you must resist! Scratching can make you bleed and ruin the tattoo. So if you get the urge to scratch, slap it instead— slapping still helps alleviate the itch without causing any damage. Applying ice can also temporarily relieve itching.*

lifetime
maintenance

The greatest and most important tip for keeping your tattoo looking its best for as long as possible is sun protection. You already know the sun can damage your skin—and while sun exposure may darken your skin, it will fade your tattoo. Have you ever seen a stuffed animal after a few years of sitting in the back window of a car? I had a black stuffed dog in the back of my car for a couple of years, and when I took it out one day, the side that had been pressed up against the window had turned a burnt orange color. That's what the sun can do to your ink!

Every time you're out in the sun, even for just a few minutes, the exposure to harmful ultraviolet rays does damage. You may not see it, and it may be so subtle that it's almost nonexistent. But every minute you spend in the sun adds up.

The best thing you can do for your tattoo (and your skin's health in general) is to make it a habit to apply sunscreen every day as part of your morning routine. Any part of your skin that isn't covered by clothing needs to be protected with sunscreen.

∽ SPF Factors and Choosing a Sunscreen

There are many levels of protection available with sunscreen and sunblock. If you're wondering what level you should use to best protect your ink, it helps to understand what those SPF numbers mean.

SPF stands for sun (or sunburn) protection factor, and the SPF number on a bottle of sunscreen indicates how well it will protect you from UVB rays, which are responsible for sunburn. So a much higher SPF would give you a much higher level of protection, right? Well, yes and no.

The number doesn't actually stand for how much protection it provides, but rather how long a period it will continue to protect you for. An SPF of 15 means that it will protect your skin from being burned 15 times longer than if you weren't wearing sunscreen. If you would normally burn in 10 minutes, you'll be safe for 150 minutes instead. Likewise, an SPF of 45 will protect you for 45 times longer.

But a higher SPF does add a *little* extra protection. A sunscreen with an SPF of 15 filters out about 93 percent of UVB rays, whereas an SPF of 30 filters out 97 percent. It doesn't get much better from there—higher SPFs can only offer a longer duration of protection.

Keep in mind, though, that this is not an exact number and even the testing done to determine SPF is very imprecise. It also does not include UVA protection, which may not burn you but still puts you at risk for skin cancer. And if you sweat or get wet, you're still going to need to reapply, no matter what SPF you're using.

∽ Sun and Indoor Tanning

How are you supposed to get a tan if you're wearing all this sunscreen? Actually, as I already mentioned, most sunscreens don't protect against UVA rays, so wearing sunscreen doesn't inhibit your ability to tan. But UVA rays aren't harmless—they're what cause the "leather skin" effect and can also lead to skin cancer.

If you must get a tan, outdoor tanning in the sun is a lot better for you than direct UV exposure in a tanning bed. Either way, make sure that you do protect yourself and your tattoo as much as possible.

> *TIP: If you like the golden look on your skin, you can always opt for a spray-on tan or bronzing lotion as long as your tattoo is fully healed. It won't do any harm to your ink at all and will still give you a healthy glow without the risk of damage to your skin or your tattoo.*

○ Touch-ups

If you're noticing that your tattoo isn't looking as bright as it used to, you can always have it touched up. That means having your artist go over the tattoo again to give it new life.

Although touch-ups can brighten faded colors, they can also thicken finer lines. Sometimes it's wise to have only the colored areas touched up and leave the outlines alone, unless they are badly blurred or faded.

If you're not able to go back to your original artist, you can always go to a different artist for the touch-up. But be aware that no matter whom you go to, you still have to pay for the work. Tattoos don't come with lifetime guarantees.

○ Your Tattoo in Twenty, Forty, Sixty Years

Unfortunately, no matter how well you take care of your tattoo, time does take its toll on all of us. Even after just five or ten years, you'll probably notice that the lines of your tattoo will spread out and fuzz a little bit. Artists know this when they do your tattoo in the first place and account for those changes by not doing too much detail or putting lines too close together. These subtle changes are most likely noticeable only to you and no one else.

Fortunately, in contrast with some of the old military tattoos from the 1950s and '60s, black ink doesn't turn blue or green over time like it used to. That was caused by the oxidation of metallic fragments contained in the inks back then. Metallic ingredients have been determined to be unsafe, and even though the FDA doesn't regulate tattoo inks, professional ink makers have stopped using ingredients they know to be hazardous. So inks should stay pretty true to their original colors through the years, although they can still fade.

As our bodies age and our skin thins out, our ink will obviously be affected. Wrinkled skin will mean a wrinkled tattoo. Skin that has stretched will stretch out the design. Weight loss and weight gain, repeated sun exposure, liver spots, and other things that come along with age can change the appearance of your tattoo. These very issues are common reasons why some people will choose not to get inked. I've had a lot of people ask me, "What will you do when you're eighty and your tattoos are faded and distorted?"

Personally, I'll still wear them with pride. If I live to be old enough for my tattoos to get wrinkled and faded, then I will have lived well. I think of lines and wrinkles as the badges of honor we earn with age. Add pictures to those lines and wrinkles, and I'll be a walking memory book of my life, my accomplishments, and the things that meant the most to me.

If you're afraid that you'll resent your ink when you get older, then it's probably not a good idea for you to get it now.

troubleshooting tattoo problems

Unfortunately, sometimes things can go wrong with a tattoo. Whether it's the artist's fault, the client's, or just "one of those things," there are occasions when a tattoo will need special attention. If you're having problems with your ink, this section can help you discover the reason and what can be done about it. Please keep in mind that this is not a substitute for a professional diagnosis or medical treatment.

✑ Bruising and/or Swelling Around a New Tattoo

It may look bad, but bruising and swelling around a new tattoo is harmless and will go away on its own. An ice pack helps with swelling, and both problems should subside in a few days. I've noticed that tattoos done in areas of thinner, more tender skin are more prone to these symptoms. Several years ago, I got a butterfly on my breast and completely panicked the next day when it looked like I had hickeys all over my boob! My artist assured me that they would go away, and they did.

✄ Cattoo Is "Weeping" Fluid and/or Ink

On the first day, and sometimes on the second day, after getting a tattoo, it's possible that you will seep clear plasma from your tattoo. This is common and normal, and can simply be washed away. It should stop on its own no later than the second day.

After that, though, a weeping tattoo—especially if the seepage contains tattoo ink—is usually a symptom of your using too much ointment or your body not liking the ointment you're using. Try cutting back on that first. It's a very common mistake, and it may eliminate the problem. Use only enough ointment to barely create a glossy finish on top of your tattoo and then dab it to remove any excess. If that doesn't work, try switching to something different.

✄ Small Red Bumps All Over the Cattoo

Little rashlike red bumps are an indication of an allergic reaction, and in the case of tattoos, it's generally a reaction to the aftercare ointment. Neosporin and similar triple antibiotic ointments are known offenders for causing a bumpy breakout, but anything can cause a reaction if your body is sensitive to it.

Stop using any ointment at all, and wash your tattoo with only very mild soap until the bumps are gone. Then begin using a different ointment or lotion until the tattoo is healed. If you break out again, keep eliminating whatever you're using until you figure it out. It's fine to just keep your tattoo clean and not put anything on it at all—it will heal just fine, although you may need a touch-up at some point if you had color loss from the bumps.

✄ Cattoo Is Flaking and Peeling Bits of Ink

Peeling and flaking are parts of the normal healing process. It's similar to the way your skin peels when you're healing from a sunburn. It's perfectly normal—and not at all harmful to your tattoo—for ink to be in those flakes of skin. That's just the dead top layer of skin. Remem-

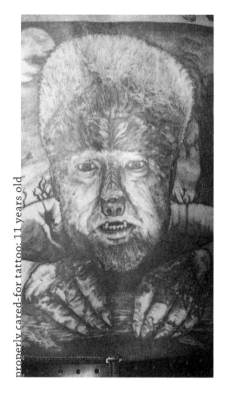

ber that your artist pushed the ink way down into the dermis, where it is nestled safely. Losing that top layer won't result in any loss of color.

If your tattoo is established and suddenly starts to peel and flake, this is likely a dermatological problem, and you should see a doctor.

"Halo" of Color Under the Skin Around the Tattoo

This effect is called a blowout, and it's usually caused by the needle having been injected too deeply or at too much of an angle, which is typically the result of inexperience on the part of the artist. It can also happen if the client's skin is very thin and not stable enough to hold the ink in place. A blowout happens when the tattoo ink "bleeds" into territory it doesn't belong in, underneath the skin. Unfortunately, there is no way to fix this problem other than covering it up with more ink, meaning that you'd have to expand your original design. If the blowout was caused by the tattooer, don't go back. You're better off finding a more experienced artist to fix it. If it was caused by unstable skin, there is a risk of it happening again, and fixing it will require great care and skill by the artist.

⨯ Raised, Swollen, and Itchy Tattoo

If your tattoo is still new and hasn't completely healed, give it time. Being slightly raised or puffy and itchy are normal signs of the stages of healing. If your tattoo is exhibiting these symptoms after two weeks or more, then this is usually a hypersensitivity (or allergic) reaction to environmental conditions.

Some people find that their tattoos get this way only on very hot, humid days. Others experience the swelling and itching only in the dead of winter when their skin is very dry. It could even be a reaction to something you ate or drank, too, and your tattoo just happens to be the place where your body is exhibiting its allergic symptoms.

These types of physical reactions are usually mild and more annoying than painful, so the best way to treat them is with ice packs, antihistamines (like Benadryl), or an anti-itch lotion (like Gold Bond). The symptoms will usually subside after a few days and won't return for a while. If it's still bothering you after you try these simple remedies, though, don't hesitate to see your doctor or dermatologist.

‿ Raised, Red, Blistered, and Oozing Only in Certain Color Areas

If you've got oozing blisters or bumps and they happen to occur only in certain areas of your tattoo—like where there's red or orange ink—this is likely an allergic reaction to the ink. Red inks and other colored pigments that have red in them are the biggest culprits for causing allergic reactions, although any color has the potential for causing hypersensitivity.

Mild reactions may subside with antihistamines, topical antibiotics, and time. But some red-ink allergies can be quite severe. Unfortunately, the only way to completely get rid of the problem is to get rid of the ink, and that's through laser removal. Severe blistering can lead to infection, so it's very important that you seek medical attention.

Since allergies can develop slowly after repeated exposure, any one of us could suddenly have a reaction to ink that never gave us problems before. It's even possible for a healed tattoo to suddenly rash out once sensitivity has developed.

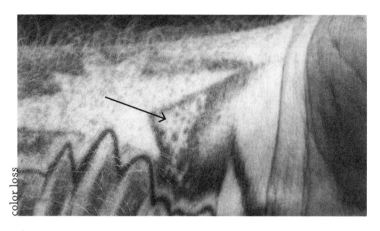

color loss

৵ Color Loss or Scarring

Once your tattoo is at least two weeks old, you can take a critical look at how well it has healed. If you see small scars or areas where a little bit of color was lost, you can have that touched up now. Most artists offer one free touch-up within a certain amount of time after you receive a tattoo.

Raised or textured scars from scabbing will soften over the next couple of months and sometimes will completely disappear. Keeping the skin supple with lotion or vitamin E oil will help with this.

Severe raised areas of scarring are called keloids. Keloids are most prominent in black people, but they can happen to anyone. Keloid scarring is caused by the body overdefending itself. It responds to the wound by building too much corrective tissue and doesn't know when to stop. Unfortunately, keloid scars don't just go away with lotions or oils and require medical intervention to remove them.

৵ Red, Hot, Swollen, Ulcerated, and Oozing Tattoo

If your tattoo has a red halo around it, feels hot to the touch, or is swollen and oozing fluids from ulcerated blisters—especially if those fluids are yellow or green in color—then you probably have an infection and need to seek immediate medical attention. Mild infections get worse fast, and staph infections can be downright deadly. Don't try to treat an infection on your own!

Important! If you're a teen whose parents don't know about your tattoo (if you got the tattoo illegally or if you know your parents simply wouldn't have allowed it), and you think you have an infection, please don't continue to hide it! If you absolutely can't go to your parents, then go to your school nurse or another adult you can trust and have the infection treated. This is really serious, and keeping your secret could cost you your life!

> *TIP: Still can't find the answer you're looking for? Don't hesitate to go back to your artist if you have concerns! They don't shut the door on you when you walk out of the studio—they take great pride in their work and want to see it well cared for, so they are more than willing to answer your questions and help you solve any problems. If you're not able to contact your original artist, just stop by any professional shop in your area. They'll be happy to help you out because they want your future business. Don't call them on the phone—they can't diagnose a problem without being able to see it.*

tattoo removal and cover-ups

If you've followed the advice in this book, it's not likely you'll regret any future tattoos you get, but you might already have one that doesn't live up to your new, higher standards. If that's the case, you're not necessarily doomed to forever walk this earth with a tacky tat. There are a couple of options.

ஒ Cover It Up

A cover-up is when you get a new tattoo over an old tattoo. It sounds simple enough, but it's actually a tricky process and requires an experienced artist to pull it off correctly. If it's not done right, residual lines and color from the preexisting tattoo will show through, which isn't a very attractive result.

There are limits as to what can be covered and how it can be covered. Depending on the size, detail, and colors of your original tattoo, an experienced cover-up artist will know what type of design and colors it will require to effectively disguise the old ink.

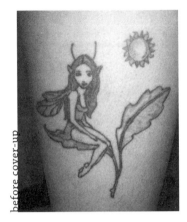
before cover-up

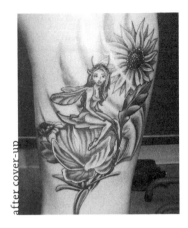
after cover-up

If you're in the market for a cover-up, search for an artist carefully. Check out their portfolios for before-and-after photos of cover-up work they've done. Can you see any evidence of the old tattoo through the new one? It may take a little extra effort to find an accomplished cover-up artist, but it will be worth it. Usually, only one old tattoo layer can be covered—if you're not happy with the cover-up, then you're stuck. This is a one-shot deal to fix up an old mistake.

If covering up the old ink is not an option and you simply want it gone, your other option is to have it removed.

> *TIP: Can a tattoo be covered with flesh-colored ink to make it blend with the skin and hide the tattoo? Unfortunately, the answer is no. Perfectly matching your skin tone with tattoo ink would be very difficult, and the old tattoo would still show through the lighter ink anyway.*

⌘ Tattoo Removal

The most common and reliable method of tattoo removal so far is through the use of lasers. The word "laser" is actually an acronym for "light amplification by stimulated emission of radiation." So using lasers to remove a tattoo involves having a very intense beam of energy, in the form of light, directed over your tattoo. The ink under the skin absorbs the light and then basically self-destructs by fragmenting into tiny particles. The cool thing about this is that it doesn't harm any live tissue surrounding the tattoo because it doesn't absorb the energy. The resulting ink particles are small enough to then be consumed and digested by the scavenger cells, which are part of the body's immune system. The whole process usually takes about two weeks after a laser treatment.

One treatment is rarely ever enough to remove an entire tattoo, but it depends on the type, color, and depth of the ink. Blues and blacks absorb the laser energy more readily and thus are more easily dispersed. Yellows and greens, on the other hand, are more stubborn and difficult to remove.

Getting laser treatments to remove a tattoo is somewhat painful—comparable to the pain of getting the original tattoo—but it doesn't drag on as long. One full session lasts only minutes. Many people describe it as feeling like being snapped repeatedly with a rubber band. If you have to get multiple sessions, you can expect a three-week break in between, to allow time for previous treatment injury to heal. During this time, you'll see that your tattoo will begin to look faded.

There are some risks associated with getting laser treatment. Although rare, it's always possible to get an infection. Two common and related risks are hyper- and hypopigmentation, which is an overabundance or a lack of melanin in the treated area, causing your skin to look either lighter or darker than its natural color. In both cases, these pigment changes can be permanent, although sometimes the skin will regain its normal color after several months.

The biggest risk, though, which has decreased with the improvement of tattoo-removal laser technology, is permanent scarring. More advanced laser removal systems do drastically reduce this risk, but it remains a plausible threat.

The biggest drawback to laser tattoo removal is probably the cost. Removing one average-size tattoo will require multiple sessions and cost

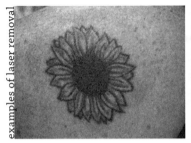
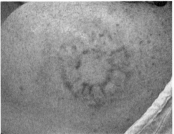

examples of laser removal

hundreds of dollars. This is why so many people opt for covering up an old tattoo rather than removing it.

If you're looking for a "middle of the road" solution, you might just get one or two laser treatments in order to fade the ink so that the cover-up allows you more options.

> *TIP: If you have a gang-related tattoo that you want removed, there are many government and private programs that can help you pay for the treatment; some even offer the service free of charge. Call your local social services department to see if there is such a program in your area.*

✿ Tattoo Removal Creams

There are several companies that offer special creams and ointments that are supposed to slowly fade a tattoo until it's completely gone. The phrase "snake oil" comes to mind when I see these products. Most of them aren't worth the price of the containers they come in. Some of them may slightly fade a new tattoo, but not significantly enough to make it worth the time, effort, and expense. If the ointments were actually caustic enough to penetrate through and destroy pigment, they would also destroy your flesh in the process. So my conclusion is that they're more useless than dangerous, since there haven't been any reports of flesh-eating creams I've heard of.

❧ Saline Injection

Saline injections are a somewhat experimental method of fading a tattoo that some artists offer clients before a cover-up. It won't remove the tattoo, but it will fade it slightly and make an easier job of covering the old ink. The artist actually "tattoos" the skin with a simple saline solution, so that the fluid is injected into the dermis where the old ink resides and flushes some of it away. It's not a fail-proof method, and very few artists offer it, but it is perfectly safe and certainly worth a try if you want to at least lighten your tattoo.

tattoo conventions

If you really want to get a feel for what the body art community is all about, consider attending a convention. Tattoo conventions are not lame geek magnets full of techie nerds discussing the latest advances in tattoo technology. Nor are they depraved, satanic, sex-orgy cult meetings. So if you're picturing either of those scenarios, you might be disappointed.

Tattoo conventions in fact draw a wide variety of people from all cultural backgrounds. The types of people you'll run into range from the curious to the heavily modified, and all are welcome.

Conventions are typically held in hotel banquet rooms or convention centers. The floors are lined with hundreds of booths, and each one will have something or someone interesting to see, whether it is an artist's booth or a retail vendor offering fun clothing or jewelry items. There's also generally a lot of side entertainment to keep people coming back for more. Some of these sideshows include live bands, fashion shows, and hook-suspension displays that may not appeal to everyone, but you can pick and choose what you do or don't attend.

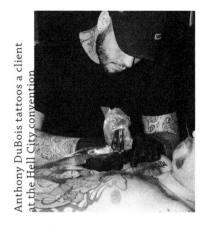

Anthony DuBois tattoos a client at the Hell City convention

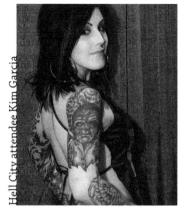

Hell City attendee Kim Garcia

The major purpose of a convention is to bring as many tattoo artists together as possible under one roof, thus providing tattooers with clientele and the visitors with artists. Attending a convention is a great way to get inked by an artist you might not normally have access to. If they live too far away or are usually too busy, you might be able to squeeze yourself into their schedule during a convention if you act quickly.

One of the best things, though, is just watching and meeting people. Lots of attendees go all out with exotic hair and clothing and will show off their most impressive tattoos and body piercings. If you like to play dress-up, a tattoo convention is the greatest place to be anyone you want to be and fit in no matter what!

Not all conventions are the same and not all of them are fabulous—I've been to a few that were actually boring. The things that usually make a convention worth attending are:

HISTORY

If a convention has been around for several years and is still going strong, that's a good indication that it has something to offer.

GUEST LIST

Great artists aren't going to waste their time attending a show that isn't

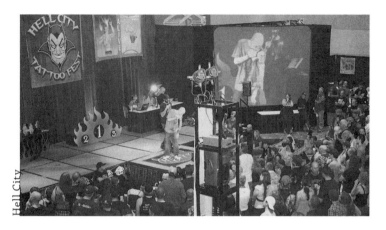

Hell City

going to give them the exposure or business they need. A convention with an impressive guest list of popular and talented artists is definitely a good sign; if it's worth it to them to attend, it will probably be worth it to you, too.

ENTERTAINMENT

Entertainment costs money, and if the purveyors of a tattoo event have the money to put into keeping their guests entertained, then they're doing something right. Bands, fashion shows, suspension exhibitions, and other "extras" make the convention a well-rounded experience.

ACCOMMODATIONS

If a tattoo event has been welcome at the same hotel or convention center for several years, then that's a good indication that the event is kept under control and in good taste. Events that bring in overly rowdy guests and stir up trouble aren't going to be invited back or be able to offer discounted room rentals to their patrons.

The best way to enjoy a tattoo convention is with a friend or group of friends. Bring plenty of money so you can get some cool souvenirs and maybe even a tattoo while you're there. Don't be afraid to approach

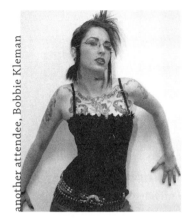

another attendee, Bobbie Kleman

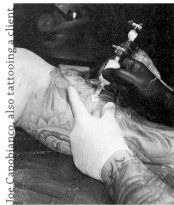

Joe Capobianco also tattooing a client

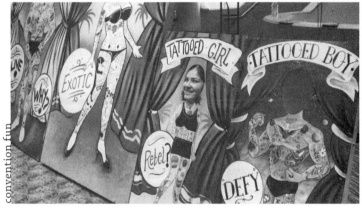

convention fun

people you don't know and ask to get a closer look at their body art—this is the place where we all like to share and meet people who appreciate our decoration. But please do be respectful; don't touch without asking permission, and ask before you take photos. And keep a close eye on your belongings—unfortunately, in every crowd there are always at least a few people who can't be trusted. The most important rule you have to follow, though, is to have fun!

tattoo FAQs

Although a lot of information has been covered at this point, there are always unanswered questions. I can't anticipate or address them all, but I will broach some of the more popular questions that I wasn't able to fit into the prior subsections.

✑ Can a Woman Get Her Breasts Tattooed If She Has Breast Implants?

Breast implants in no way hinder a woman's ability to get tattooed. The tattoo needle does not penetrate far enough to get anywhere near where the implants are, so no, it will not "pop" them.

✑ Does Hair Growth Hurt a Tattoo?

If you get a tattoo in an area where hair will grow back afterward, it will not harm your tattoo at all. It can, however, change the appearance of the tattoo if the hair is thick or long. If you don't like the look of hair growing through or over your tattoo, you can keep it shaved or waxed, but that's a personal choice. But don't shave until your tattoo is at least a week old and there are no scabs or flakes. Don't wax for at least a month, and don't use chemical hair removers for three months.

What's a Cramp Stamp?

I hate the term "tramp stamp," which refers to lower-back tattoos that are most common among women. It's derogatory and insulting, and I hate it when women use it when referring to their own lower-back tattoos. I don't know when or where it got started or who started it, but using this term is no different from propagating any other stereotype. Where a woman decides to get a tattoo is her business.

Can I Still Get a Tattoo If I'm Sick?

If you've got a cold or the flu, please have consideration for your artist and reschedule your appointment. Not only will it be more difficult for your body to heal if you're already sick, but your artist doesn't need you spreading your germs to them and putting them out of work.

Is It True That You Can't Get an Epidural If You Have a Lower-Back Tattoo?

No and yes. Here's the thing. There is absolutely no evidence to support the claim that an epidural puncture through a tattoo could be hazardous. Someone came up with the idea (it may have even been a doctor, I don't know) that pushing the epidural needle through a tattoo could introduce toxic ink into the spine and harm the patient. Now, if that actually could happen, I could certainly see the cause for concern. The fact is, though, that the probability of ink transference and the possibility of the ink being toxic are both so minimal that it's about as likely as your odds of being trampled by an elephant. I suppose it *could* happen!

I'm not a doctor, but there have been many doctors who have stood up and refuted this claim about lumbar tattoos and epidurals; there are also those who don't dismiss the claim. So what does this mean for you?

Ask your doctor. Until there is actual scientific research, there isn't really any proof one way or another, and doctors simply have to make a decision based on their own medical expertise and experience. But in my ten years of writing about body art, I haven't seen a single story of anyone being hurt from getting an epidural with a lower-back tattoo.

✧ Is It Okay to Get a Tattoo If I'm Pregnant?

Pregnant women shouldn't get tattoos for two main reasons. One is that your body needs to heal from getting a tattoo, and your body has to then make a decision—heal the tattoo or take care of the baby. One or the other will usually get the short end of the stick, and neither situation is good. Draining your energy resources to heal a tattoo takes away from your unborn child, but if the tattoo doesn't heal and you end up with an infection, that will also hurt your baby and you.

The second reason is that in the event that you have a reaction to the ink, end up with an infection, or (worst-case scenario) contract a disease like hepatitis from a dirty needle, you will pass on that danger to your unborn child. It's just not worth the risk, and you only have to wait a few months before you can safely get tattooed.

✧ Is It Okay to Get Tattooed If I'm Breastfeeding?

Just as with pregnancy, when a woman is nursing a baby she passes on to her child anything that goes into her own body. If you are nursing and get an infection or a disease from a bad tattoo, you risk delivering unhealthy milk to your child. Unlike with pregnancy, though, this is more of a judgment call. An artist won't necessarily refuse to tattoo you if you're nursing, but they may try to discourage you. The difference is that if you do develop a physical ailment, you can always stop nursing, but remember: Not all ailments are apparent from the onset.

✧ Can I Get a Tattoo If I'm on My Period?

There's no reason you *can't* get a tattoo if you're on your period, but you might not want to. Some women just don't feel good or are more sensitive to pain during this time, so getting poked repeatedly with needles might not be an appealing idea. Plus, if you take aspirin-based pain relievers to deal with cramps, they could cause bleeding complications while you're getting the tattoo. If your period sneaks up on you when you have a tattoo appointment, just call your artist as soon as possible to reschedule if you need to.

‿ How Can I Become a Tattoo Artist?

Becoming a tattoo artist requires time, patience, and dedication. If you didn't read the section of this book on the difference between scratchers and professionals, make sure you do. You'll need to find a professional tattoo artist willing to mentor you and pass on the tricks of the trade— that's called an apprenticeship. Apprenticeships aren't easy to find, but if you are persistent you'll find one.

It's not necessary—or desirable—to know how to tattoo before finding an apprenticeship; your mentor will teach you everything you need to know in that regard. But it is important for you to have either natural talent or fine-arts training and be able to show real aptitude when it comes to drawing and using colors.

A full apprenticeship that will take you to the point of being able to go it alone should take at least two years. Anything less than that, and you're probably being cheated out of important training and supervision. Some apprenticeships last up to five years—it all depends on the artist and the one being trained.

Tattoo schools do exist, but they're really not well respected. They charge several hundred dollars for a weekend of training and then throw you to the wolves. There is no way you can learn everything you need to know during a weekend crash course, and most tattoo shop employers are not going to be impressed if your only experience is from a tattoo school. Opening your own shop is simply not an option for newcomers to the trade; it's a business failure just waiting to happen.

piercing guns versus piercing needles

There are two main ways you can be pierced. One is with the gun—a squeeze unit that uses the actual jewelry to pierce the skin; the other is with a piercing needle, which makes a hole that the jewelry is then pushed through. When you go to jewelry shops or department stores, they use the squeeze gun method. When you go to a tattoo shop, they use a needle. What's the difference between these two methods, and which is better?

❧ The Piercing Gun

Let's examine the gun method more thoroughly first. The gun itself is made primarily of plastic, and the mechanism inside it is made of metal. The mechanism has a cutout that juts out and surrounds the ear, holding the earring post and backing separate but aligned. When the trigger is squeezed, it activates a metal shaft inside the gun and forces the post through the skin and then through the hole that attaches the back to the post. It's relatively quick, and since the jewelry insertion is part of the process, once it's in, you're ready to go. Sounds good, right?

Most people think so, and that's why a lot of people get their ears pierced this way. But then these same people wonder why their piercings won't heal and why they get so many infections from them. Well, I can tell you why.

First of all, the piercing gun isn't sterile. The jewelry itself comes from a blister pack that is clean, but the gun can't be sterilized. Because it's made of plastic, it would require intense heat that the plastic parts wouldn't be able to handle. So, to "clean" the gun, a piercing practitioner will wipe it down with rubbing alcohol or a similar antiseptic. In case you didn't know this already, antiseptics don't kill blood-borne pathogens, the really harmful germs that carry HIV and hepatitis. And they also don't kill most regular bacteria with just a few swipes—even Clorox kitchen wipes recommend wiping for thirty seconds to kill 99 percent of germs. Would you feel safe if your surgeon wiped down his tools with just antiseptic right after using them on a person with hepatitis C? I don't think so! Don't be fooled into thinking that the gun is clean just because they give it a few swipes with an alcohol pad.

Another problem with the piercing gun is the way it forces the jewelry through the skin. Another term for it would be "penetrating trauma." Even though the tip of the post might be pointed, it's still pushing a relatively dull object through the skin by force. And then it squeezes the jewelry stud and the back so tightly around the skin that it can hardly get any air, which doesn't help the healing process. This traumatic blow and pressure to the skin cause undue swelling and pain, and then the lack of air only makes it worse and can lead to infection.

One of the biggest problems with the guns—and what finally woke me up as to how awful they are—is the malfunction rate. They're not complicated pieces of machinery, but they get "hung up" in the middle of a piercing quite often. The mechanism gets jammed easily. When my five-year-old daughter was getting her ears pierced (in the days before I knew better), she had to deal with the practitioner attempting to unjam the gun by twisting, pulling, and squeezing the trigger a few more times, all while it was still attached to her ear. Not a pleasant experience. Now fourteen, my daughter still remembers that day vividly.

If that's not enough reason to be wary of the piercing gun, here's another: Even the jewelry itself poses a problem with healing. The stud and post style (with the butterfly back) cover so much surface area that it's difficult to clean and becomes a breeding ground for bacteria. When sebum manages to seep out of the wound hole, it gets caked in and around the back of the stud and all around the butterfly back. There are so many tiny surfaces that there is really no way to effectively clean it without removing the jewelry completely. Bacteria gets trapped inside all those nooks and crannies of dried blood and sebum and begins to spread, and the next thing you know, you've got a nice infection.

TIP: The piercing gun was designed for use on earlobes only. Using it anywhere else or for any other kind of procedure is illegal in many states. The risk of infection or spreading disease is even greater when the gun has been used on ear or nose cartilage, which still takes place in many stores. Imagine getting pierced with the gun after it had been up someone's nose—yuck!

Last but not least, getting your ears pierced with a gun means you're not in the hands of a professional. The salespeople have about fifteen minutes' worth of training (one of them told me they practiced on teddy bears for about fifteen hours) before they're sent out to start poking people. They expect the gun to do all the work, and crooked, misaligned piercings happen all the time. Then, to make matters worse, they give you "cleansing solution" that contains just about the worst ingredients you can possibly use on a new piercing. The antiseptic properties of these solutions do more harm than good—they may kill some bacteria, but they also inhibit the growth of new, healthy tissue. The harshness of these cleansers can actually cause more irritation and pain than the piercing itself. Finally, to

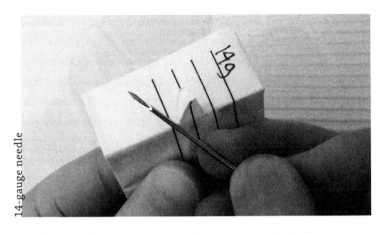

14-gauge needle

top it off, they tell you to rotate your jewelry during the healing process, which only causes more irritation and introduces bacteria. Left untreated, this can lead to a serious infection.

Granted, a lot of these are worst-case scenarios, and plenty of people get pierced with the gun without incident, but why take the chance when there is something so much better out there?

∾ The Piercing Needle

Let's now see how the piercing needle works in contrast with the gun. The needle is a long, slender surgical instrument with a very sharp, beveled point, and it's made of surgical stainless steel. There is no machine to control the needle—only the piercer's hands. Piercing needles come in many sizes to accommodate different piercings in different locations of the body. It is approved for use anywhere on the body and through all kinds of tissue. But how does it really compare?

Instead of just being wiped down with some antiseptic, piercing needles are autoclave sterilized, which means all bacteria and blood-borne pathogens are destroyed. All other tools, such as clamps, corks, cleansers, and marking pens, are either autoclavable or disposable. That's not to say nothing could ever go wrong or that mistakes are never made, but your chances of being exposed to bacteria are almost nonexistent.

Now let's examine the method by which the needle actually pierces the skin. Instead of forcing the blunt post of a stud through the skin, the needle gradually slices through the skin. That may *sound* graphic, but it's actually very gentle in comparison with the gun method. The point of the needle is inserted first, and the pressure increases incrementally as it passes through the tissue. Instead of being forced through in less than a second, it actually takes several seconds for the needle to be carefully guided through the skin. This is much less traumatic to the skin and a lot less painful than punching through it with a jewelry post.

One of the biggest differences between the needle and the gun is the malfunction rate. The needle has no mechanisms that can potentially fail, so it has zero risk of breaking down in the middle of your piercing. The only thing that could possibly "malfunction" is the piercer—and that brings us to the next point of comparison.

When you go to a licensed studio to get pierced by an employee, you are not being pierced by a salesperson with limited instruction. Piercers go through extensive training before they are allowed to work on real people in a professional shop. They learn about sterilization, anatomy, associated risks, metal allergies, jewelry types, and aftercare, as well as proper piercing procedures. They do dozens of supervised piercings and have to prove themselves before they can start piercing people on their own. They don't just pierce you and shove you out the door. If something goes wrong with your piercing or your jewelry, they're trained to answer your questions and help you fix the problem. Given my daughter's experience, I'd only ever entrust my appendages to a real piercer.

So what about the jewelry? You won't see any post-and-stud jewelry with butterfly backings at a piercing shop. Instead you'll see barbells, CBRs (captive bead rings), labret studs, talons, claws, plugs, and earlets—to mention just a few of the styles of body jewelry. Not all of these styles are appropriate for new or small-gauge piercings, but your piercer is qualified to suggest what kind of jewelry is best for whatever procedure you are getting. Several metal types are available if you have nickel sensitivity or other metal allergies. Basic CBRs and barbells are usually recommended for new piercings and are so much better for your skin—they allow easier access for cleaning, let the skin breathe, don't encourage bacterial growth, and are overall more conducive to successful healing. And healing is our last point of comparison.

Professional piercers are trained in the best methods of aftercare for their clients. They know which products work and which ones don't and can make the best recommendation on how to clean and care for your new piercing. Some of them even send you home with the products you'll need, or at least sell them at the shop. And the majority of piercers agree that antiseptic solutions are just about the worst thing you can put on a new piercing, so they won't be sending you home with any of that stuff! My piercer sends me home with a bottle of Satin therapeutic skin cleanser and a little plastic baggie full of sea salt, along with a fully detailed instructional sheet on how to use them.

Again, I want to stress that not all tattoo and piercing shops are as clean and sterile as they should be, and not all piercers are as professional as they ought to be. But in most cases, you're in much better hands going the licensed shop/professional piercer/needle route than the jewelry kiosk/untrained salesperson/gun route. Some state health departments are already cracking down on the use of the gun, and many of us would love to see it banned completely. It's just not worth the risk, especially when there is a much safer alternative available.

∞ What About Kids?

My personal gripe on the needle-versus-gun issue is the fact that I could take my ten-year-old to the mall and let their untrained salesperson use an unsanitary gun to pierce her ears, but most tattoo shops won't pierce someone that young. In some states, it's illegal, and sometimes it's just company policy. Usually, I would advise parents in this situation to talk to their child's pediatrician. Many of them will pierce your child, and it's legal for them to do it regardless of age because they're licensed physicians. However, I ran into a snag there myself—my pediatrician would do the piercing, but he doesn't use the needle. He uses the disposable squeeze-gun method, which is cleaner than the traditional gun but still just as traumatic, and still uses post-and-stud jewelry. So, after a year of wanting her ears pierced, my daughter is still waiting.

I want to help her get pierced, because if I don't find a way to pierce her safely, she's probably going to rebel before she's old enough and come home sporting a safety pin that was jabbed through by one of her friends on a dare. If you're a parent in the same situation, I still say ask your pediatrician first. If that's a no-go, then you may need to take your kid somewhere—even out of state—where the minimum age is lower or nonexistent. Either that or simply wait and hope they don't make an unsafe decision on their own before they're old enough to be pierced properly.

> *TIP:* If you're a minor who wants a piercing and you can't—due to either local laws or your parents saying no way—please don't pierce yourself or let a friend do it. It really can be very dangerous; people have actually died from piercing infections, and many have gotten very sick. It's just not worth the risk when in just a few years you'll be old enough to get all the piercings you want—safely.

fear and pain

CHAPTER 27

How much does getting a piercing hurt? That's usually the first thing a person wants to know before they get one. It's a fair question, but not one that's easy to answer. It depends on where you're getting the piercing, how much tissue the needle has to go through, and what your personal pain threshold is. All of these factors vary from person to person and can make even identical piercings a very different experience.

Piercing through cartilage tends to hurt more than it does through soft tissue, but even that is subjective. My industrial was really painful, but my tragus barely hurt at all—and they're both cartilage piercings. The dermal anchors I got through the soft tissue of my chest were pretty intense, whereas my eyebrow piercing was very easy. Piercings that I had found painful, others have told me were not bad at all, and vice versa. It's difficult to say whether *you* will find a particular piercing very painful or not.

One thing I can say in regard to the pain that comes with piercings is that it's over very quickly. It's not like sitting through an hour-long tattoo session, being poked repeatedly. It's one or two pokes in a matter of seconds, a bit of a squeeze to insert the jewelry, and you're done. The overall intensity may be more than that of getting poked with a tattoo needle, but most of us can handle even harsh pain for a few seconds. A few of my piercings did make my eyes water, but that was the worst of it.

And just like people who get tattoos, people who get piercings go back for more and more. If it was so difficult to endure the procedure, only masochists would be returning for further torture. I don't think the throngs of people lining up at the piercing shops are all masochists—I know I'm certainly not. And yet I've gotten eighteen piercings and still have plans for more in the future. I may not *enjoy* the pain of the process, but the results are worth it in the end.

TIP: Ever heard the phrase "bite the bullet"? Well, there's a lot of truth in that advice—having some gum to chew on, or even a pencil to bite down on, during the temporary pain of the piercing can really help! I wouldn't recommend biting down on an actual bullet, though.

Relief Before It Even Starts

You can use a numbing gel, like the kind made for a sore tooth, to help take the edge off an oral piercing. It starts working pretty fast but also wears off quickly, which is okay because the piercing doesn't take that long to begin with. Skin surface piercings are a little trickier. There are creams available, like EMLA, which are pretty expensive and take at least a half hour to take effect. That's a lot of trouble to go through for a thirty-second piercing. Some creams also affect the elasticity of the skin, which is more of a problem with tattooing but still can present a challenge when trying to place a piercing exactly right. Discuss your pain management desires with your piercer first; some of them already use numbing products they are comfortable with, while others may suggest you bring something with you.

TIP: Many body art enthusiasts feel that body piercing is a rite-of-passage experience that shouldn't be cheated through the use of pain inhibitors. It's a very quick process, and there is a natural "high" you get when your endorphins rush in to protect you from the pain. It's that euphoric moment that secures a spiritual bond between you and the new jewelry you wear—your prize for bravery and strength of will. Do you really want to reach the destination without experiencing the journey?

ᏮFear of Needles or Blood

If you have a pronounced fear of needles, getting a piercing can be an intimidating experience. Unlike tattoo needles, which barely break the skin, piercing needles actually go through several layers of tissue and are physically comparable to an injection. That's probably not much comfort, but the only real encouragement I can give you in this case is that you don't have to watch and it's over very quickly.

I suppose it's a mind-over-matter kind of thing. If you really want the piercing, you're just going to have to overcome your fears for a few seconds—grin and bear it, so to speak. Piercers are usually very gentle and sympathetic to clients with these fears. They will do everything within their power to make you comfortable and provide an experience that is as stress-free as possible. Since this is a voluntary procedure, it's a little easier to face. After all, the outcome is going to give you something you want. Just keep the end results in your mind's eye and remember why you're doing this in the first place!

As far as blood goes, most piercings produce very little, but there is usually at least a drop or two. If that's going to make you ill, you might want to ask your piercer to clean you up thoroughly and be sure that you're not actively bleeding before they let you see your new piercing. But, really, it's not going to gush. Again, it becomes a challenge of the mind to overcome it, but jumping these emotional hurdles can actually help you conquer your fears. Bearing in mind, again, that it's completely voluntary and has positive results will get you through it.

> *TIP:* Feeling faint? It could have nothing to do with the pain or blood, but rather occur because your blood sugar levels dropped too quickly, in which case a couple big gulps of soda or some pure sugar can get you back up to normal. Lie down flat and take calming breaths until the dizziness subsides.

the risks of
body piercing

While body piercings in and of themselves are not inherently dangerous, there are associated risks that you need to be aware of. Many piercings are subject to minor issues. It's important that you understand the potential problems that could occur as a result of body piercing, but it's even better to know how to prevent problems or treat them before they become serious.

Of course, your first line of defense against serious problems is making sure that you go to an accredited, experienced, and qualified piercer for all procedures. But even if everything is done as cleanly and safely as it can possibly be, problems can still arise. Many piercings are subject to minor infection. Migration and rejection, which can result in scarring, are common problems, especially with surface piercings. Mild irritation and small bumps happen frequently, particularly with cartilage piercings. For most of us, these issues are trivial and not enough to prevent us from getting pierced. Chapter 38 can help you to deal with many of these minor inconveniences, which usually go away after a short time. But sometimes it's too high a price to pay for a piece of jewelry.

‿ Preexisting Health Issues

Because piercings are small and not permanent like tattoos, it's easy to have a laid-back attitude about them. For most of us, that's okay; I can decide purely on a whim to go get something pierced and not really give it a second thought. If I decide I don't like it or if it isn't comfortable, I'll simply take it out—no big deal. But for some people, it is a big deal.

In October 2002, seventeen-year-old Daniel Hindle Anderson entered Body Poppers in Sheffield, United Kingdom, with his girlfriend, Naomi. The two planned to get pierced together, so Naomi got her eyebrow pierced, and then Daniel got a lip ring.

Daniel was born with a congenital heart defect called tricuspid atresia, which prevents the blood from flowing to the lungs properly to collect and disperse oxygen. Although he'd had two lifesaving surgeries when he was young and had lived a normal and healthy life since then, people with this heart defect have to see a cardiologist regularly for the rest of their lives to monitor their heart functionality, because it's possible for things to go wrong at any point during their life span. They are also at an increased risk for endocarditis, which is an infection of the heart valves, and many of them have to take antibiotics just for a routine dental visit.

At the time, there were no laws in Sheffield that regulated any kind of body piercing practices, so it's difficult to know for sure what happened, but a few days after Daniel got his piercing he began to feel ill. His condition worsened, and two doctors were called out to see him during the next couple of weeks. The first doctor misdiagnosed him as having food poisoning, but the second realized there was something more serious going on and had Dan sent to the hospital. He was transferred to the ICU after being diagnosed with septicemia, a very advanced infection of the blood more commonly known as blood poisoning. This was just two weeks after he had gotten the lip piercing. The doctors agreed with Daniel's mother, Christina Anderson, that the piercing was probably the source of the initial infection.

Daniel continued to fight the infection for another six weeks, but in the end, it was just too much for his heart to take. He died on December 21, 2002, of circulatory failure. An inquest into his death was conducted, and although the court did rule that Daniel's death was a tragic accident, the coroner, Christopher Dorries, admitted that cardiologists needed to make their patients clearly aware of the risks of body piercings. He said, "Those vulnerable to infection need to understand that this is not just fusty old adults trying to stop their fun. There can be very real risks."

> "Dan was outgoing, well-liked, good-natured, had a lovely sense of humor, and always [wore] a smile. [He] was also an extremely bright and intelligent young man; an accomplished musician with a vast eclectic record collection. Dan was on the cusp of his adult life, ready to embrace the world and everything that the world had to offer. The world is indeed a poorer place without Dan. The irreplaceable void that losing Dan has created for myself, his siblings, family members, and all his many friends is heartbreakingly vast. There are no words to convey how much we love and miss [him]. Dan will live in our hearts and our memories forever."
>   —CHRISTINA ANDERSON

The bottom line of this sad story is that Dan made a decision he never would have made if he had been fully informed. He wasn't aware that getting a "simple" piercing—something millions of people have done without incident—could cost him his life. And even though the piercing shop wasn't found to be at fault in Dan's case, with or without a heart condition, piercings can be dangerous. (See Chapter 38 for Zeke Wheeler's story.)

Daniel's family continues to campaign to this day for stricter regulations, which still don't include an age minimum. Christina Anderson told me that as of 2004, body piercing practices in the U.K. remain dangerously unregulated. There is no statutory age limit for ear piercing or cosmetic body piercing within England and Wales. However, London Boroughs have used licensing powers to impose license conditions relating to the age of the client. These regulations are subject to review in 2010, at which time they will hopefully improve to protect even more young people. In the interim, Christina Anderson personally spreads the word about body piercing safety through school workshops and a website built in Dan's honor. She wisely says, "Knowledge is power and we should never underestimate this fact. Empowering our young people to make choices that are more informed is something we all have a responsibility and an obligation to do."

If you have a preexisting condition that could, in any way, make a mild infection life-threatening, getting pierced becomes a very big deal. Piercings—even ones done professionally—are often subject to minor infections. They can appear out of nowhere and be much worse than you think. Daniel and his family had no idea how badly his body was being ravaged by infection; he had told his mother he simply felt "off."

In a similarly traumatic story, Stephanie Edington from Indiana had her nipples pierced for her eighteenth birthday on August 29, 2006. A few weeks later, her nipples became red and sore and began to seep fluid. On October 14, Stephanie was admitted to the Indiana University Medical Center with an infection. Her condition progressed to the point where a mastectomy of her left breast and the removal of all flesh up to her collarbone were the only ways to save her life from the deadly necrotizing fasciitis (gas gangrene) that was destroying her body.

The piercing shop and the piercing itself were not found to be at fault for Stephanie's exposure to the bacteria, but the piercing wound was the perfect entry point when she did somehow come into contact with it later. To make matters worse, Stephanie is diabetic, which is a condition that slows the body's ability to heal and makes it more susceptible to complications.

If you believe you may be at risk, talk to your doctor before getting pierced and get their advice. If you decide to get the piercing, watch it very closely and seek medical help at the first sign of anything abnormal. (See Chapter 38 to learn the signs of infection.)

⤾ Risk of Disease

When you are pierced in a professional shop, by a professional piercing artist, and in a properly sterile environment, your risk of being exposed to blood-borne pathogens (like hepatitis or HIV) is slim to none. However, that doesn't mean it could never happen. Piercers are human, and humans make mistakes. There is always a minimal risk both you and your artist share, but Standard Precautions—the sterile chain of events set by the CDC to be followed by all professional piercers—gives everyone involved great protection against disease exposure.

If you try to pierce yourself, have a friend do it, or go to "some guy" who does it out of his house really cheap, that shield of protection offered by Standard Precautions goes out the window; you have nothing to guard yourself against blood-borne pathogens. Yes, many people get lucky and don't get sick from unsafe piercings. But do you really want to play roulette with your life and hope you're one of the lucky ones?

⤾ Piercings in the Workplace

Finding a good job can be difficult for anyone, but throw in a few body piercings, and your search becomes even more complicated. Despite the growing acceptance of body art in mainstream society, there are still a lot of employers out there who will think you're not good enough to work for their company if you're pierced anywhere but your earlobes. For guys, even the lobes may be too much.

Even if company policy doesn't require that you remove your piercings, some companies expect their employees to cover them up with a bandage. Truth be told, I think the bandage thing is ridiculous, and I have a hard time believing that some company heads actually think that it looks more professional and less offensive than a piece of jewelry.

I'd be the first person to applaud you for turning your back on such companies and being your own person. But, when it comes down to it, we all need money—and for that we need to work. Sometimes you have to pick your battles, and choosing a piercing over a paying job is kind of silly. At times, though, it is possible to have your cake and eat it, too—see Chapter 30 to find out how a retainer can help you make your piercing virtually invisible.

∽ Donating Blood and Plasma

If you're a regular blood and/or plasma donor, you'll need to consider this as well. In many states, you can't donate if you've gotten a body piercing within the last twelve months. This restriction exists so that any blood-borne illness you might have been exposed to will have had time to show up. To avoid allowing tainted blood into the donor pool, they make you wait.

The good news, though, is that some states are relaxing this restriction if you can prove you got your piercing at a licensed, state-approved studio. Since they know these studios follow Standard Precautions, the odds of your carrying a disease after being pierced there are so slim that they consider it safe. You'll need to check with your local Red Cross to find out what your local laws are and whether or not you're still under the twelve-month restriction.

effects of alcohol and drugs

Before getting pierced, you may be tempted to self-medicate a bit to calm your nerves or ease the pain of the procedure. Or maybe the desire to get pierced in the first place came about after having a few drinks or hanging out with friends. But drugs and alcohol aren't going to make getting pierced any easier, and they may prevent you from getting pierced at all. Consider how they affect both your body and your cognitive thinking.

✷ No Sober, No Service

If you like to party, that's your business. But if you party before you walk into a shop for a piercing, it becomes their business. If you appear to be under the influence of any kind of alcohol or mind-altering drugs, they will not pierce you.

Why? Because the first thing you have to do before you can get pierced is sign a legal document that gives the piercer permission to puncture you and states that you agree to their terms. If you are not of sound mind, you can't legally agree to anything, and your signature would be worthless. You have to be sober to sign the paperwork.

In addition to that, drinking alcohol thins out your blood by decreasing the coagulation "stickiness" of the blood cells for about twenty-four hours after consumption. Thinner blood and lack of coagulation mean heavier bleeding, which isn't a good start toward a happy, healthy piercing.

৶ Prescription Drugs

Any prescription drug that has a blood-thinning effect should be avoided if possible. Talk with your doctor to see if it's safe to skip your medication for a day to get a piercing.

Other than that, there aren't too many prescriptions that interfere with the piercing itself, but they may interfere with your ability to heal afterward. Even antibiotics can kill the good bacteria you need to heal your piercing. Be sure to tell your piercer about any prescription drugs you are taking, so they can tell you whether it could hinder your healing ability.

Also, prescription drugs you may be taking might be an indication of a medical condition that could make getting pierced very dangerous. It's important that you are honest with your piercer about your health status and any prescription medication you are taking.

৶ Over-the-Counter (OTC) Medications

Even some seemingly harmless OTC drugs can harm more than help. Aspirin or aspirin-containing products thin out your blood just like alcohol and should be avoided for at least twenty-four hours before you get pierced. If you need to take a pain reliever in the meantime, it's best to stick to acetaminophen (like Tylenol).

types of body jewelry

The first thing you should know about body piercings is the type of jewelry used. You won't find the typical stud-and-post jewelry or dangles from French hooks. Body jewelry is a style all its own, and it's designed to be more conducive to healing and comfort.

ᴄᴑ CBRs (also known as BCRs)

The CBR, or captive bead ring, is the closest thing to the traditional "hoop" earring. It's a circular piece of metal with a small space between the two ends. That space is used to insert the jewelry, and then it's closed by placing a small bead in between the space. The sides of the bead are dimpled so that it "pops" in place and holds tight to secure the ring and keep it from coming off. In many European countries, the CBR is known as a BCR, to stand for "ball closure ring," which is the same concept.

ᴄᴑ Barbells

The barbell is so named because it resembles the kind of barbell that weightlifters use. A bar, which can vary in length, is closed on each end

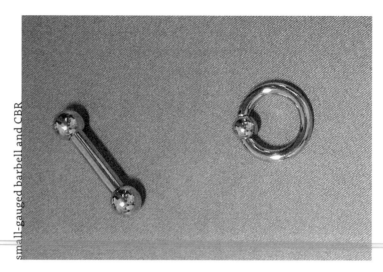

small-gauged barbell and CBR

with a ball. Sometimes both ball ends can be removed, and sometimes one comes off and the other is stationary. Either way, at least one ball is unscrewed from the end to insert the jewelry, and then the ball is replaced to secure the jewelry in the piercing.

Barbells aren't always straight. Curved barbells are also sometimes called bananabells because of their shape. Circular barbells are actually a little more horseshoe-shaped than round.

> *TIP: Barbells can be either internally or externally threaded, which describes how the ball end screws into the end of the bar. "Externally threaded" means that the end of the bar is threaded and goes inside the threaded ball. "Internally threaded" means that the bar is smooth on the outside but threaded inside. The ball end has a tiny threaded nub on the end that screws into the end of the bar. Internally threaded barbells are considered superior because a threaded bar end going through raw tissue can cause damage. Also, internally threaded ball ends are stronger and more secure than the external ones.*

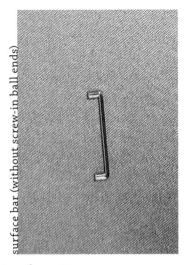
surface bar (without screw-in ball ends)

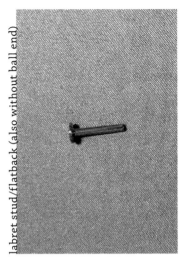
labret stud/flatback (also without ball end)

✑ Surface Bars

Surface bars are specially designed for surface piercings. They look very similar to regular barbells, except that the ends are bent up at a ninety-degree angle so that they stick directly out of the skin instead of entering and exiting at an angle. This design greatly reduces any pulling or tension on the piercing due to natural movement. The advent of surface bars has greatly improved the success rate of many surface piercings.

✑ Labret Studs/Flatbacks

Labret studs are small bars that have two different ends—a ball on one end for outside the mouth and a flat disc on the back for inside the mouth. The purpose of the flat disc, as opposed to a ball, is to keep the jewelry flush against the inside of the mouth and prevent the gums and teeth from being irritated by contact. Even though a labret is actually a specific type of piercing, any piercing that uses this type of jewelry is usually just referred to as a labret stud.

There are other types of jewelry with flat discs on the back, but they're much longer and can come in a variety of shapes and styles, such as spikes and other decorative ends.

TIP: Despite the effort to reduce irritation through the use of a flatback, the metal discs can still harm teeth and gums. Since the discs are removable and usually come in two sizes, it's best to always get the smallest size available to minimize rubbing as much as possible. Some companies are even starting to offer biocompatible silicone or plastic backs, so you might want to check into that as well.

✎ Nostril Screws, Fish Tails, and Nose Bones

Nostril screws and fish tails are sometimes confused, but they're basically the same thing with one small difference. They both give the appearance of a "stud," meaning that only a small shape or gem is visible on the outside, similar to a traditional stud earring. But instead of being held in place with a butterfly back, they're held in place by the shape of the bar. A nostril screw is already bent into a curved flat shape that is easy to insert into the piercing. But since it's not custom fit to size, there may be some additional movement you didn't bargain for, which is why I personally prefer a fish tail. It comes with a straight bar that is bendable and can be made to best fit your piercing.

Nose bones are shorter than nostril screws and fish tails, and what holds them in place is a small, stationary ball on the end. The problem with nose bones is that the piercing has to be forced open even wider to accommodate the ball at the end. Cartilage doesn't respond well to being forced in this way; it can be quite painful and lead to prolonged irritation after the jewelry is inserted. If you want to wear a nose bone, it's best that you don't plan to change your jewelry very often.

✎ Earlets, Eyelets, and Tunnels

Designed for enlarged piercing holes, earlets and eyelets are the same thing with different names: small, open cylinders with either one or both ends flared out to hold them in place. If only one end is flared, then the other is held in place with an o-ring. If both ends are flared, that means

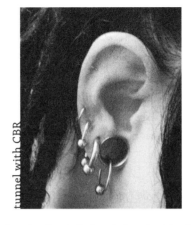
tunnel with CBR

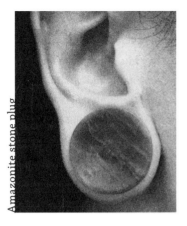
Amazonite stone plug

the piercing hole has to be stretched even larger to allow one end of the tube to pass through. This risks damage to the piercing, so the kind with only one flared end is preferable.

Flesh tunnels are even better than earlets, especially if you prefer the double-flange look and don't want to wear o-rings. One flared end of a tunnel will unscrew to allow for easy insertion. Once it's screwed back into place, you can't even tell that it isn't all one piece.

∾ Plugs

Plugs are exactly what they sound like. They serve as a stopper to fill the hole of an enlarged piercing. In contrast with earlets and tunnels, they're solid and come in a variety of shapes and styles. Some are completely smooth and held in place with o-rings on both sides. Some have one flanged end and some have both. Depending on the size of the piercing and the material the plug is made of, they can be very heavy and not comfortable to wear for long periods of time.

∾ Claws, Talons, and Spirals

Claws and talons are pretty much the same thing, except that claws curve more than talons do. They are curved, tapered bars—the bottom starts out small and pointed, and the gauge size slowly graduates through the

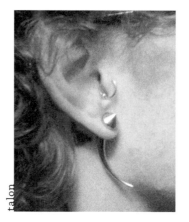

talon

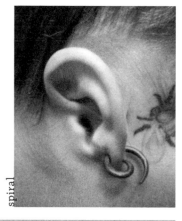

spiral

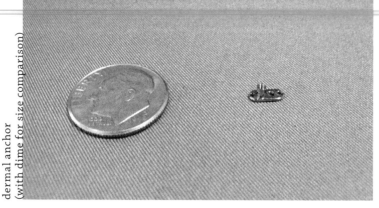

dermal anchor
(with dime for size comparison)

length of the bar. They're usually worn in stretched-lobe piercings and can even be used to encourage a gradual stretch by wearing a size slightly larger than your current piercing gauge. They're held in place with o-rings on each side of the lobe.

Spirals are similar in that they're tapered bars, but instead of just curving they can be quite ornate, with several curves and twists. My favorite earrings that I have are a set of swan spirals, which do resemble a swanlike shape. Sometimes spirals also need to be held in place with o-rings, but if they spiral enough or are heavy enough on the bottom, they may hold in place on their own.

✎ Tusks

Tusks aren't quite like they sound—they aren't made to stick out of your mouth like walrus or elephant tusks. Actually, they're worn in the nose—through the septum, to be exact. The long bar is usually tapered on both ends and is worn so that it goes through the septum and comes out each nostril. They're usually held in place with o-rings.

Some tusks are short and small, while others are very long and large and can actually cover the nostril passages. If you happen to like breathing through your nose, you might want to avoid this particular adornment.

✎ Dermal Anchors

Typically made of implant-grade titanium, dermal anchors are placed under the skin and have a small, threaded end that sticks out in order to attach a gem that lays flat against the surface. The anchor—the part that stabilizes the whole piercing underneath the skin—is made in such a way that it actually encourages the tissue to surround it as it heals, making it more or less a permanent part of the body. That's why the anchor will sometimes have small holes in it.

✎ Retainers and No-C-Ums

Retainers are designed to keep a piercing hole occupied without being visible. Usually made of acrylic, Lucite, or some other form of plastic, they're not typically meant for long-term wear because they aren't as biocompatible as other materials. But when you need to hide a piercing for work or a special occasion, these are a great option over removing the piercing and taking the chance that it'll close up on you.

> *TIP: Retainers are great, but just as they're not meant for long-term wear, they're also not meant for new, unhealed piercings. New piercings need to have metal jewelry to allow for proper healing, and retainers shouldn't be used until the*

piercing is at least three months old; changing it out too soon could lead to an infection. So, unfortunately, if you're already in a school or job that doesn't allow piercings, getting it done over the weekend or a holiday isn't going to allow sufficient time for healing before you can use a retainer to hide it.

✎ How Body Jewelry Size Is Measured

There are three terms you need to acquaint yourself with when it comes to choosing the right-size jewelry: gauge, length, and diameter.

The gauge of a piece of jewelry is how thick it is—that thickness has to correspond with the size of your piercing hole. Get it too small, and your hole will shrink up; get it too big, and you'll be forced to stretch your piercing, which can be painful if done without the proper tools.

The smallest size that body jewelry is usually available in is 20-gauge, which is approximately eight-tenths of a millimeter in thickness. Gauge sizes go down in number as the thickness increases, and body jewelry gauges come only in even numbers, so the next size up from a 20-gauge is an 18. From there, it counts down in even numbers from 16- to 0-gauge, which is about eight and one-quarter millimeters thick. After 0, it goes to 00, 000, and 0000, before they finally give up and start referring to sizes by measurement. After 0000, it goes to a half inch, and then there are several incremental sizes from there on up to two inches or even bigger.

The length of a piece of jewelry matters only if there is a bar involved, and the length is the measurement of the bar itself. One-quarter inch is usually the smallest size, and then it goes up in incremental lengths from there. The smaller the gauge, the smaller you can make the length.

Last but not least, you'll need to know the diameter if you're wearing a CBR or something else with a circular shape. The diameter is the distance from one side of the circle to the other, in a straight line. If the diameter is too small, it could be too snug against your skin, which can make it rub and pull—not a pleasant feeling. If the diameter is too big, the jewelry will stick out too far from your skin surface and could even get caught

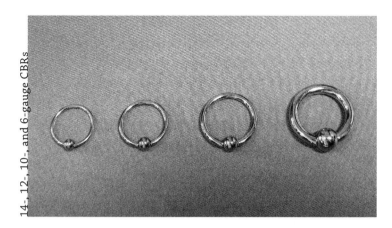

on things—another unpleasant experience. So it's important to get the diameter right.

Really small circles and rings are also going to have smaller gauges—thicker-gauge jewelry has to be made into larger diameters. A 20-gauge CBR can be as tiny as a quarter inch in diameter, while a 6-gauge has to be at least half an inch or more.

✎ Materials Used to Make Body Jewelry

Body jewelry is made from many different materials. Some of those materials are highly biocompatible and highly accepted by almost everyone. Others are lower quality, more prone to allergic reactions, or meant only for temporary wear. It's important to know the difference, because a lot of piercing infections and other problems are caused by the jewelry itself or because it was used improperly.

SURGICAL STAINLESS STEEL (SSS)

In the United States, this is the most common starter jewelry material for any new piercing. It's durable yet inexpensive and is biologically accepted by most people. There are different grades of SSS, though, and it's always best to wear only the highest grade available, which is 316L (the L stands for "low carbon"). Most body jewelry suppliers have now started supplying only 316LVM SSS items, which are a step above 316L because the metal is vacuum melted. The result of that process, in addition to creating the highest available grade of SSS for body jewelry, is a surface that's practically flawless, which makes reaction and irritation rates even lower.

However, SSS still contains nickel—the main culprit when it comes to allergic reactions to jewelry—and it still can cause a problem for sensitive skin types. In fact, many European countries have banned the use of SSS entirely for new piercings because of this, and allow only niobium or titanium starter jewelry. The reason SSS causes less problems than other nickel-containing metals is that it releases the nickel at a much slower and lower rate.

> *TIP:* *Nickel hypersensitivity can develop at any time, even if you never had a problem with it before. Nickel exposure is cumulative, so the longer you're exposed to it, the more it builds up in your body. For some people, this becomes a problem at a point when their bodies decide they can't handle the nickel anymore and begin to react to even minor contact with it.*

NIOBIUM

Niobium is a metal that's harder and denser than SSS. The risk of scratches in the surface (which can harbor bacteria) is extremely low, and the presence of nickel is almost nil. Niobium passes the European nickel exposure laws, so it can be used as starter jewelry.

Niobium used to be a very popular choice because it can be turned different colors by anodizing it, which is a really cool process. The metal is dipped in an electrolyte solution, which makes it vulnerable to electricity. Then it's exposed to an electrical current and, depending on the voltage it's charged with, it changes to one of many different possible colors. Niobium, for a long time, was the only jewelry metal available in black, until the recent introduction of Blackline/PVD.

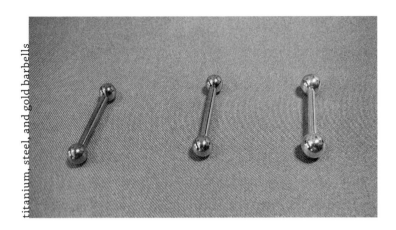

titanium, steel, and gold barbells

TITANIUM

Titanium is by far the most durable and biocompatible metal out there. It's been used in the medical field for years to make pins and plates and replacement joints for surgical patients. It's more expensive than SSS, but definitely worth it if you wear large-gauge jewelry (titanium is half the weight of steel) or have nickel hypersensitivity. Titanium contains the lowest possible amount of nickel and is biologically well accepted by almost everyone.

Titanium jewelry comes in a natural, shiny silver tone or can be anodized to create different colors, just like niobium. And more recently, it can also go through a process called physical vapor deposition, or PVD, which turns it black.

BLACKLINE/PVD

Blackline is one of the more common lines of body jewelry that has been treated with PVD. It's a complicated process, but it basically means that a titanium nitride coating has been bonded to the base material (usually SSS or titanium) to create a hard, biocompatible coating that gives the jewelry a rich black appearance. It's wear-resistant and has been approved for use in the surgical field for over twenty years, although it's a new addition to the body jewelry realm.

SILVER

Most people think of sterling silver as being pure, but it's actually not. Silver in its purest form would be too soft and light to wear as jewelry. Sterling is classified as .925, meaning that it's 92.5 percent pure silver. That leaves 7.5 percent of the metal to contain other alloys, such as nickel, platinum, or copper. What is used for that other 7.5 percent can be the difference between a quality piece and one that is no better than cheap costume jewelry.

In addition to containing other metals, some silver jewelry isn't just sterling silver. Because silver is prone to tarnishing—which can color your skin—a lot of it is coated with a rhodium electroplating to prevent tarnishing. Chipped electroplating can be harmful to the body, so silver should never be used for new piercings. Once they're healed, silver is okay to use as long as you don't have any reactions to it.

GOLD

Gold pretty much has the same problem as silver in that the more pure the metal is, the softer it becomes, making it prone to nicks and scratches. Harder grades of gold contain impurities and metal alloys that are not bio-friendly. So if you like gold, wait until your piercing is healed, and then it's always best to go for the highest grade possible. Just keep a close watch on it for scratches and clean your jewelry regularly.

PLASTICS

Body jewelry and its accessories are available in a wide variety of plastic-based materials, each one usually serving a particular purpose based on its properties. Acrylic, Lucite, PTFE (short for polytetrafluoroethylene), silicone, nylon, and resin are just a handful of the different types of plastics used by body jewelry designers.

Acrylic jewelry is popular for its wide variety of colors, light weight, and low cost, but it is not designed for long-term use. Acrylic can't be autoclave sterilized because the heat would destroy it, but it also can't

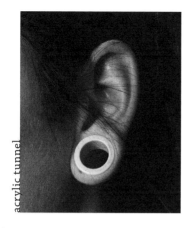

acrylic tunnel

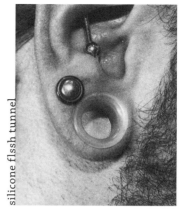

silicone flssh tunnel

be soaked in alcohol because alcohol breaks it down. It shatters under pressure, which is why a lot of people have ended up swallowing bits of their tongue rings after chomping down on the acrylic ball end by accident. Acrylic plugs suffocate your piercing and prevent the skin from being able to breathe; this is okay for short periods of time but can be detrimental if worn for more than a day. If you're going to the club for a night and you have a healed piercing, then acrylic is fine for the evening, but be sure to take it out as soon as the night is over.

Lucite—closely related to acrylic—is popular because its clear, transparent quality makes it practically invisible against the skin, making it an optimal material for retainer jewelry. But it comes with the same biocompatibility problems as acrylic, so it's also recommended only for short-term wear. It's a great option if you need to hide a piercing for work, as long as you switch back to your normal jewelry at the end of the day.

PTFE is more commonly known as Teflon. Yup, it's the same stuff used to coat nonstick pots and pans and even some clothing lines. But it's also very bio-friendly and has a long list of benefits when used as body jewelry. In contrast with acrylic, PTFE can be autoclave sterilized. It's flexible and chemically inert, which means it doesn't react to anything. Its surface is so smooth that it is almost completely friction- and abrasion-free, which means that it won't cause irritation as it moves around underneath the skin. It also doesn't suffocate the skin like acrylic and can be worn long-term without incident.

Tygon and PTFE are generally preferred for use in surface piercings. Because the strands are flexible and can be cut to length, they provide the most customizable fit, which is very important to reduce the risk of migration and rejection. Although both materials are inert and therefore biocompatible, Tygon tubing is considered superior to PTFE because it can be internally threaded, which is the higher standard.

A lot of piercers prefer to use Tygon or PTFE over surface bars, but that's more of a personal choice. Because the tubes or strands have to be manually threaded, it does require a practiced hand to secure the ends properly.

Monofilament nylon is very similar to PTFE and is generally used for retainer jewelry. It usually comes as a plain straight or bent strand that just slides into the piercing hole to occupy the space temporarily. It should be used only in healed piercings, simply because the jewelry shouldn't be changed to any retainer until it's healed.

> *TIP:* You may have heard that there are some concerns about the safety of PTFE. It's a valid issue when dealing with Teflon at high temperatures because it releases toxic fumes. This is not known to be a problem with PTFE body jewelry or any PTFE at room or body temperature, and it is still considered biologically safe.

Silicone is actually superior to acrylic in that it has the same advantages—it's lightweight and comes in different colors. But surgical-grade silicone is very biocompatible and thus approved for long-term wear. It doesn't shatter under pressure and can withstand high heat, so it can be autoclave sterilized. The disadvantage is that it doesn't come in as many jewelry styles, so it's just used to make plugs and earlets, as well as accessories like o-rings and ball-end covers.

Fimo jewelry is made from a claylike substance, but it's actually

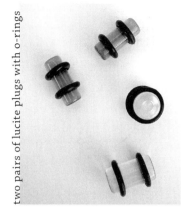
two pairs of lucite plugs with o-rings

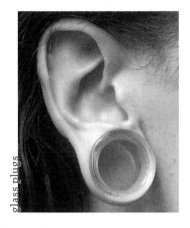
glass plugs

a polymer plastic. It's used to make plugs and tunnels and can come in a great variety of colors and designs. Unfortunately, it's not very bio-friendly, and a lot of people have problems wearing it, even short-term.

There are many other plastic-based materials that can be made into body jewelry. There's always something new popping up as jewelry makers discover new things to work with and technological advances are made. If you want to wear something you're not familiar with, it's best to check with your piercer to see if it is okay for long-term use or should be saved for special occasions only.

GLASS

Pyrex is the most common brand name of a material known as borosilicate glass. This is the kind of glass that's used for body jewelry because it's more durable and can withstand the heat of autoclave sterilization.

Glass ball ends are great accessories to metal balls, but they can also be used to make jewelry pieces of their own. Plugs, tunnels, tapers, and claws are just a few examples of the shapes that can be formed using glass. The disadvantage is that large-gauge glass jewelry can be very heavy. It should be worn only in healed piercings. Due to its weight, it's not usually recommended for long-term wear, but it is biologically friendly as long as it's not pulling or causing strain on your piercing.

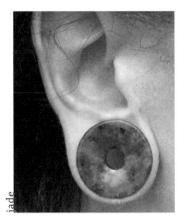

jade

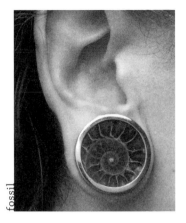

fossil

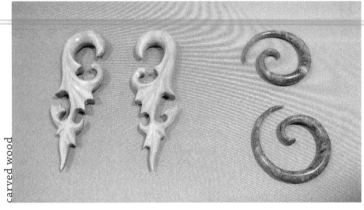

carved wood

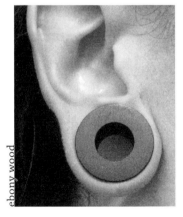

ebony wood

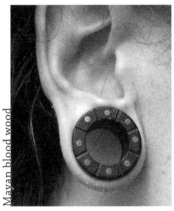

Mayan blood wood

ORGANICS

Beautiful body jewelry can be made from organic materials such as wood, bone, horn, stone, and even porcupine quills! The same rules pretty much apply to all of them. They're okay for short-term use in healed piercings only. If anything should happen to the jewelry to cause a scratch, crack, or any other kind of damage, it should be discarded.

Organics can't be autoclave sterilized, but some of them, particularly wood, have very specific cleaning instructions. It's important that you follow the instructions carefully, or you could accidentally damage the jewelry.

Even this isn't a complete list of all the types of jewelry available, and there's no doubt that more materials and styles will be introduced over time. The key is to do your homework before trying anything new and make sure anything you put in your body is clean and safe.

types of piercings

If you want a piercing but aren't sure what to get, there are a lot of options for you to choose from. The human body is a veritable pincushion and can be pierced just about anywhere you want. Granted, some locations are more convenient than others, which is why some piercings are so popular they even have names. This section will cover the most common body piercings and what you should know about them before you decide to get one.

⤮ Ear Piercings

LOBE

The earlobe has been pierced for centuries, on both men and women. The lobe is by far the easiest place on the body to pierce. It's soft and pliable, and doesn't contain any major arteries but has sufficient blood flow, which aids healing.

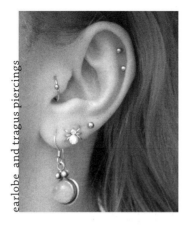

earlobe and tragus piercings

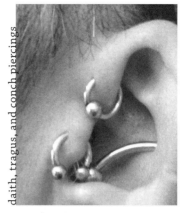

daith, tragus, and conch piercings

Typically, earlobes are pierced with a 14- or 12-gauge needle and then adorned with a matching-gauge CBR or circular barbell.

TRAGUS

The tragus is a thick chunk of cartilage in the center of the ear, but it's not as painful to pierce as you might anticipate, because it's a softer cartilage. It should be pierced with a CBR or circular barbell because they make keeping the piercing clean a lot easier. After it's healed, you can switch to a mini curved barbell if you'd like. Tragus piercings should start out at no smaller than 14-gauge to reduce the risk of migration.

> *TIP: Some people have reported hearing a popping sound in their ear while having their tragus pierced. If that happens to you, it's not an indication of any damage; it's just the sound of the needle breaking the skin. Since it's happening so close to the eardrum, it seems a lot louder to you than it actually is.*

DAITH

A daith piercing goes through the protruding fold of cartilage just above the tragus that follows the natural outline of the ear, which is anatomically

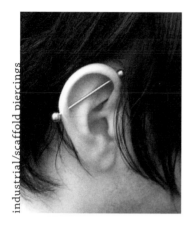

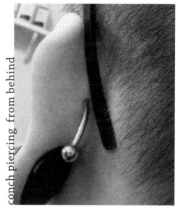

referred to as "crus of helix." This area is made of softer cartilage like the tragus, so it's not usually a terribly painful place to pierce. Recommended starter jewelry for this piercing is a 14- or 12-gauge CBR or circular barbell. It can be changed to a small curved barbell once it's healed.

ROOK

A rook piercing is inserted through the cartilage protuberance just above where a daith would go. It's a very thick bit of cartilage for most people, and this cartilage is much harder and thicker than that of the tragus or crus of helix. Recommended starter jewelry is a 16- or 14-gauge CBR or circular barbell. A small curved barbell can be inserted once it's healed.

INDUSTRIAL/SCAFFOLD

An industrial (known in Europe as a scaffold) is a fun piercing because it can be done so many ways with a variety of barbells. The standard industrial consists of an extra-long straight barbell that runs mostly horizontally, from one side of the ear to the other. The piercings are actually inserted through the helix, or rim, of the outer ear. But this piercing can also deviate from the standard method. Anytime two or more piercings of the ear are connected with a single, extra-long bar—whether it's straight, twisted, or bent—it is still considered an industrial.

It's important that you only connect piercings that were made for a particular barbell. Using a straight bar to connect two older holes that were originally meant for a CBR will put painful tension on the piercing holes. Industrial piercings should start out with a 14- or 12-gauge industrial bar that is even longer than needed, to account for swelling.

HELIX/RIM

If you follow the outer curve of your ear down to the lobe, you'll notice that it's folded inward. That's called the helix. It's a large span of cartilage, and any single piercing that occupies space along this line—even if you decide to put twenty rings all along that outer fold—is called a helix piercing. Recommended starter jewelry is a 14- or 12-gauge CBR or curved barbell.

CONCH

Your conch is the large, concave area in the center of your outer ear. A single piercing through this area is thus appropriately named a conch piercing. The conch is also a convenient place, besides the lobe, to wear enlarged jewelry like plugs or tunnels. But cartilage piercings should never be stretched; instead, a large-gauge conch piercing would need to be done with a dermal punch.

Unless you're having your conch gauged up, typical recommended jewelry for a normal conch piercing is a 14- or 12-gauge CBR or curved barbell.

TIP: The greatest risk associated with ear cartilage piercings is an infection called perichondritis, in which pus builds up between the layers of skin that surround the cartilage. If left untreated for too long, the infection can destroy the tissue by cutting off the flow of blood, which can leave you with a permanently damaged ear.

ORBITAL AND ANTI-

An orbital isn't a specific piercing of the ear, but can refer to anywhere on the ear where a single CBR penetrates the ear with both sides of the circle, making the ring orbit the ear like rings orbiting a planet. Lobe orbitals, conch orbitals, and helix orbitals are all possible.

The prefix "anti-" is used to describe an area that is opposite the part of the ear that follows the prefix. So, an anti-tragus is a piercing directly opposite the tragus. An anti-helix is a piercing opposite the helix. These terms also refer to their anatomical counterparts.

∽ Facial Piercings

BRIDGE/ERL

Given the name Erl for the first man known to get this piercing, this is more commonly known as a bridge, which is actually a misnomer. An Erl is a horizontal piercing that spans the top of the nose directly between the eyes. Anatomically, your bridge is actually much lower than this; the area between the eyes is called the nasion. Technically, it qualifies as a surface piercing, but for all intents and purposes I'm listing it here as a more common facial piercing because it doesn't have quite as high a rejection rate as most surface piercings, due to the presence of extra flesh in this area. If your skin is very tight and thin at the nasion, then it's a risky piercing because the chance of rejection is higher.

It may look like a simple piercing, but an Erl actually requires a piercer with a practiced hand and a good eye. It has to be positioned to follow the lines of the eyes and face, not just the nose, so it doesn't make your entire face look lopsided.

Keep in mind that you probably come in contact with your bridge more than you think you do. Rubbing your eyes, washing your face, wearing glasses, putting on makeup—you may find an Erl very inconvenient once you get it.

A straight barbell should never be used for a bridge piercing because it would cause too much tension at the entry and exit points. A Tygon

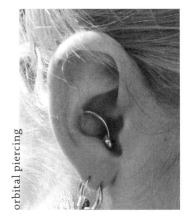

orbital piercing

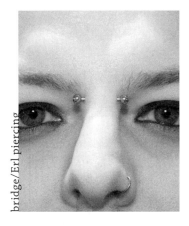

bridge/Erl piercing

bar or a small curved barbell are the best options for this piercing. The weight of a CBR could actually encourage migration, even though it does normally allow for easier cleaning and care.

> *TIP: An Erl piercing will not make you cross-eyed. You shouldn't even notice it unless you purposely cross your eyes. If the ball ends are too big or the bar too long, you may catch glimpses in your peripherals. If it bothers you, see your piercer and have your jewelry changed.*

EYEBROW

A piercing through the eyebrow, like the bridge, is technically a surface piercing. But because there is ample, soft flesh that is easy to pinch, it's not difficult to get a good, deep placement. The more tissue it can go through, the less apt your body is to reject it.

The brow can be pierced once or multiple times, vertically or horizontally. I don't recommend that the brow itself be pierced unless you don't have any eyebrow hair. The hairs can easily become ingrown or irritate the piercing, so it's best to pierce just above or below the brow line. Even then, you might have some issues with eyebrow hairs from time to time.

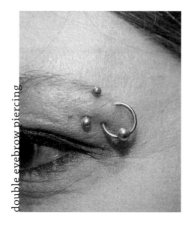
double eyebrow piercing

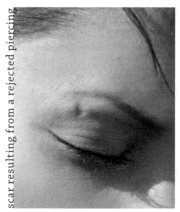
scar resulting from a rejected piercing

I have found that I have to keep my brows plucked away from the entry and exit points of my piercing to prevent problems. A few years ago, I got a nasty bump and couldn't figure out why it was so irritated. When I was shaping my brows one day, I discovered that one hair had managed to wriggle its way up inside the piercing hole. One little hair can really cause a lot of trouble!

Recommended starter jewelry is a 14- or 12-gauge CBR, curved or circular barbell, or Tygon bar. Charms are not recommended for this piercing, even when healed, because the weight can encourage migration and rejection.

> *TIP: Some piercers will claim that freehand piercing is superior to using clamps to hold the tissue in place. There is nothing to substantiate this, and the use of clamps does not mean your piercer is inexperienced. It's more personal preference than anything, and both methods can produce acceptable results as long as the piercer knows what he/she is doing.*

NOSTRIL

The nostril is actually very unique in its structure because it's soft and pliable but also complex. Your nostril is made up of thin cartilage, four

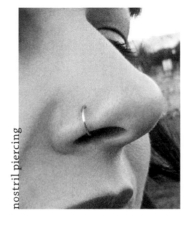

nostril piercing

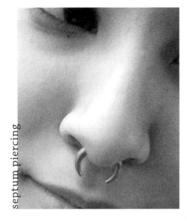

septum piercing

muscle groups, fatty tissue, blood vessels, and nerves. The delicate nature of the nostril makes it highly resistant to being pierced, but with patience and care you can usually convince it to calm down and accept its new occupant.

You may think that the nostril has to be pierced in the supra-alar crease, which is that little indent between the bulbous part of the nose and the trunk. But this is actually not the best placement, because dirt, oils, and dead skin cells tend to collect there on a lot of people. Healing a nostril piercing is difficult enough without having that working against you as well. The best placement is along the more stable alar sidewall, which is the rounded area below the crease.

The best starter jewelry for the nostril is a 16- or 14-gauge CBR. I know, a lot of people don't like the look of the ring in their nose and want to start out with a nostril screw. But nostril screws just don't allow for easy cleaning and proper healing. They move around a lot and can be a source of irritation to a new piercing. If you insist on a nostril screw, you'll need to be extra careful with your piercing.

SEPTUM

A septum piercing doesn't actually penetrate your septum, which is made of hard cartilage and would be very painful to pierce. If you put your thumb and forefinger in your nostrils and squeeze toward the middle, you'll feel

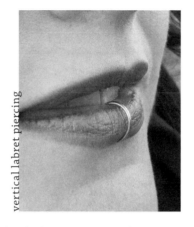

vertical labret piercing

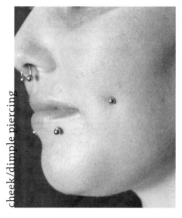

cheek/dimple piercing

the thick, spongy tissue that separates your right and left nostril holes—the medial crural footplate. Above that, you'll feel the thick cartilage of the septum. But if you pull down on the footplate and squeeze a little harder, right between those two areas, you'll find what is referred to as the "sweet spot" by many piercers. That thin, fibrous area between the footplate and the septum is what is actually punctured for a septum piercing.

A septum piercing should be started at no smaller than 14-gauge (although a 12-gauge would probably be even better) and use a CBR or circular barbell. The advantage of wearing a circular barbell is that if you need to hide the piercing, it can be flipped upside down, placing one end of the barbell inside each nostril. It's a great option if you don't want to remove the piercing, especially when it's new.

VERTICAL LABRET AND JESTRUM

Both of these piercings are vertical piercings through the lip—the vertical labret, the more common of the two, is through the bottom lip; the jestrum is through the top lip. Both of them go directly through the center of the lip, in line with the philtrum, which is that little indent between your nose and upper lip.

Both of these are the best lip piercings you can get because they don't go inside the mouth at all, so there's no oral piercing complications. After having severe gum issues because of my standard labret (see page 160), I was forced to remove it. But I really loved that piercing and missed seeing it, so I decided to give a vertical labret a try. I was really pleased with how painless it was and how easily it healed. I absolutely love it—even more than I loved my labret.

Make sure your piercer knows what they're doing, because the alignment is crucial. A crooked piercing will make your whole mouth look wrong. Because it's such a shallow lip piercing, a ring or circular barbell would protrude too much. Standard jewelry for both piercings is a small curved barbell, anywhere between 16- and 12-gauge, so both ball ends rest on the outer edge of the lip.

I'm not sure this is the best piercing for people with extremely thin lips, though, unless you can find jewelry short enough to prevent it from sticking out too far at the ends. The jewelry should be snug to create the proper effect.

> *NOTE: The next five facial piercings are actually part oral piercings as well, because the back of the piercing is inside the mouth. These combination piercings have an extra difficulty factor when it comes to healing because they require two kinds of aftercare and come with two sets of potential problems.*

CHEEK/DIMPLE

Cheek or dimple piercings are usually done in pairs—one on each side of the face. They can be placed inside a natural dimple or be used to create the illusion of a dimple because of the indent that is created by the ball end.

This type of piercing requires a very experienced piercer because if it's not done properly, things can go very badly. You're dealing with major muscle groups that control the function of your entire mouth, and there are also large blood vessels in the cheeks. In addition to that, your piercer has to watch out for your parotid gland, which is the largest of your salivary glands and is responsible for much of your ability to break down food and swallow.

It should be noted that cheek piercings leave big scars if you take them out. Even the holes may remain visible for a while. Once the holes heal up, the scars can be quite noticeable for many years. Considering this is valuable facial real estate we're talking about here, you might want to give this piercing serious thought first if you're bothered by scars.

A long labret stud is used for this piercing, usually somewhere between 16- and 12-gauge. The size of the ball is important with this piercing, too, to create the right dimple effect. If you think the ball ends are too small or too big, just tell your piercer and he/she can change them out for you.

MEDUSA AND LABRET

A medusa piercing goes horizontally through the philtrum, that little dimple above the center of your upper lip. The only part of the piercing that's visible is the ball end nestled in the philtrum, which is a nice look. The labret is pretty much the same thing, but it goes under the center of the bottom lip.

Because they both use a labret stud, that means a flat disc is on the inside of your mouth and has the risk of coming in contact with your teeth and gums. It's really important to have an experienced piercer for this one, because it has to be placed just right in order to not cause gum or tooth damage. Unfortunately, even the best of piercers sometimes can't make this one work. That happened to me.

My piercer did the absolute best he could to get my labret aligned properly, which he probably did, but what he didn't account for was my uncontrollable urge to "play" with my piercing. I felt the disc there and couldn't resist rubbing it back and forth against my gums. As a result, I started having problems with my gums and had to take it out before I did real damage. Some people have problems with a labret or medusa when it's no fault of their own or their piercer's—it just happens.

Both the medusa and the labret should be pierced with a 16- or

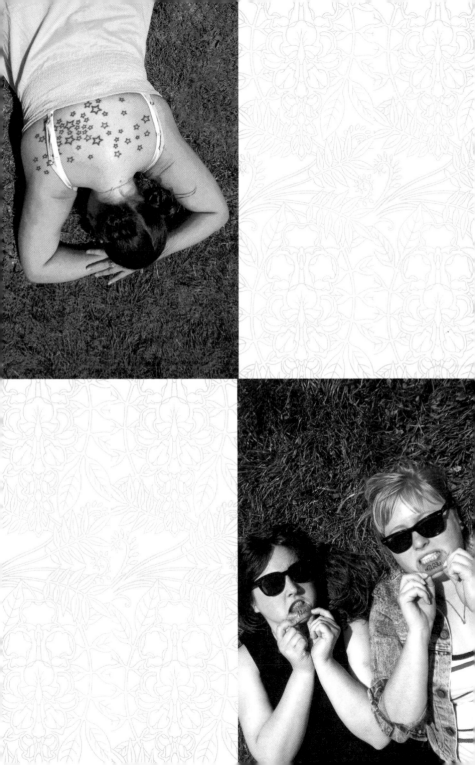

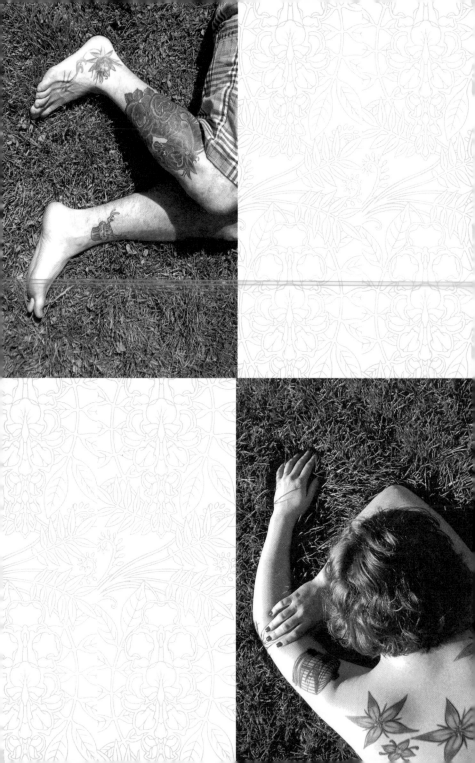

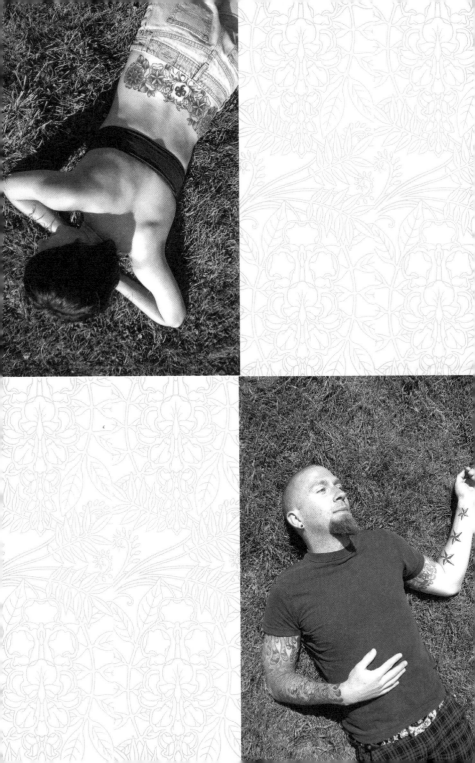

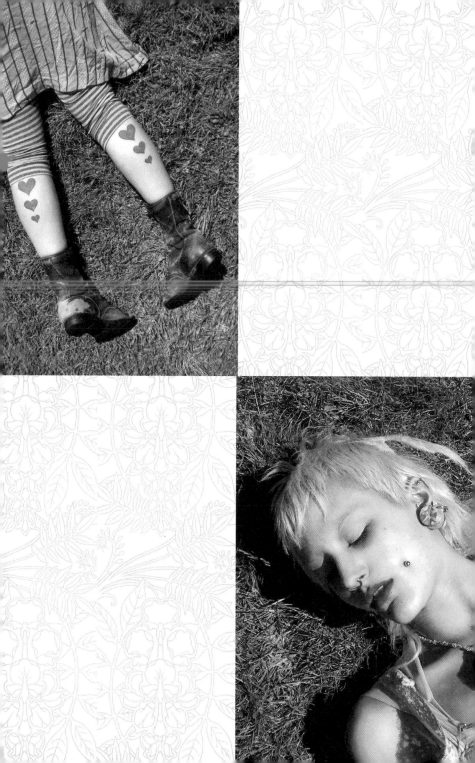

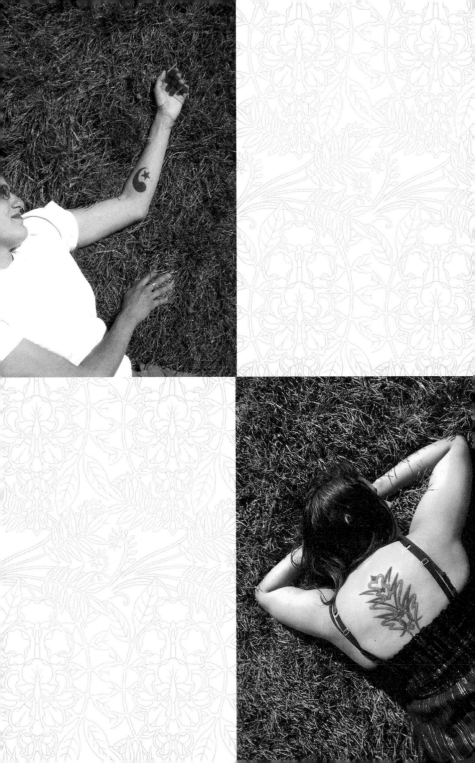

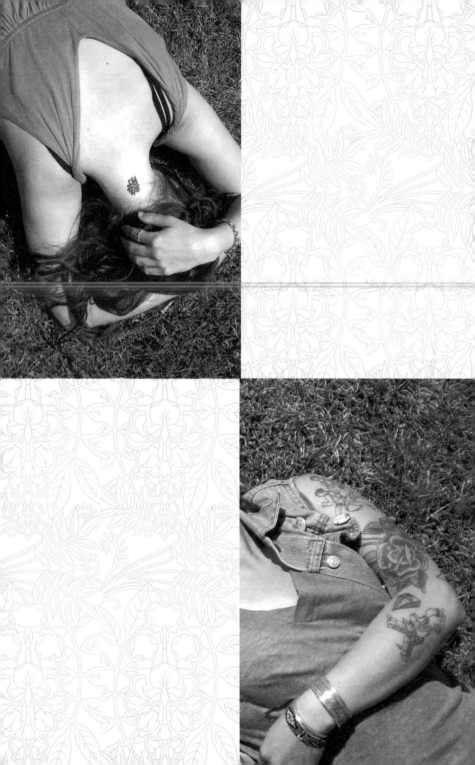

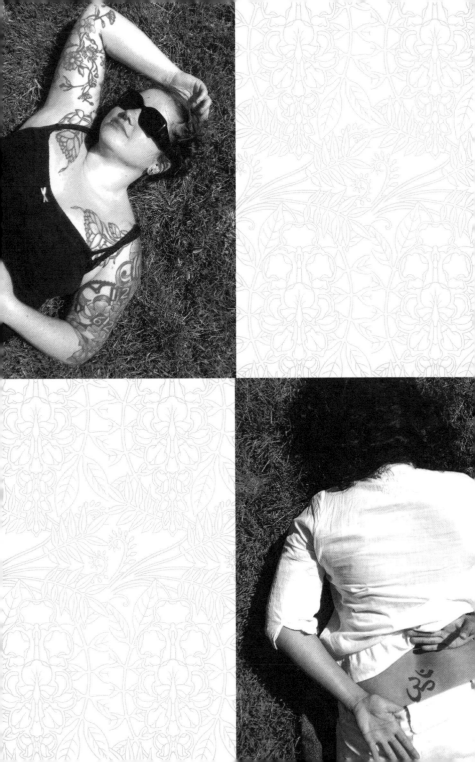

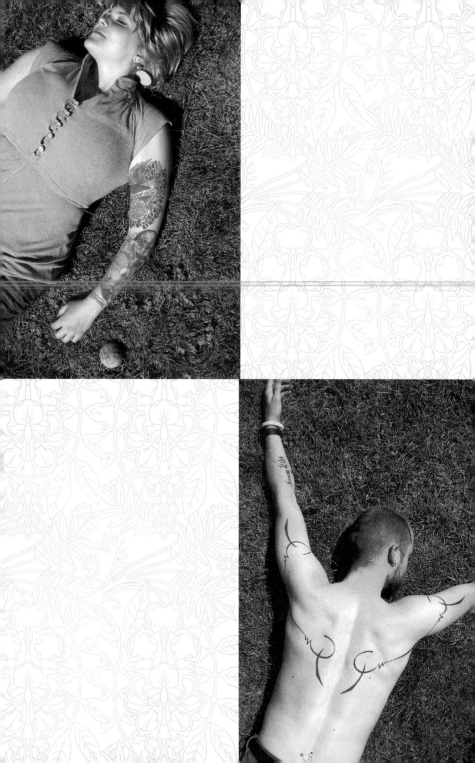

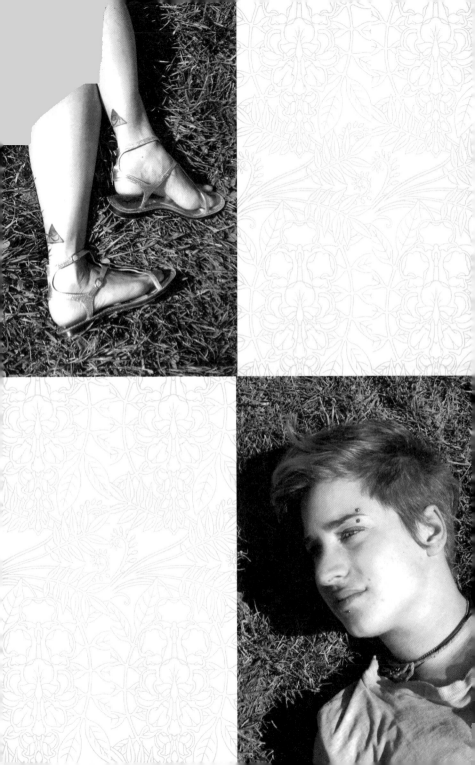

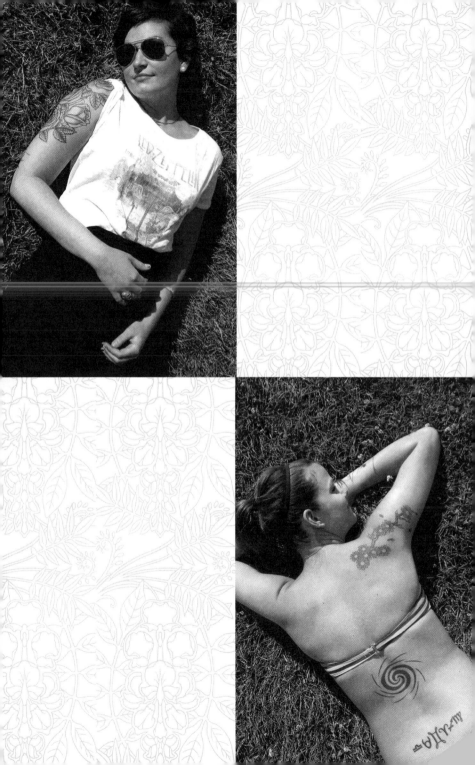

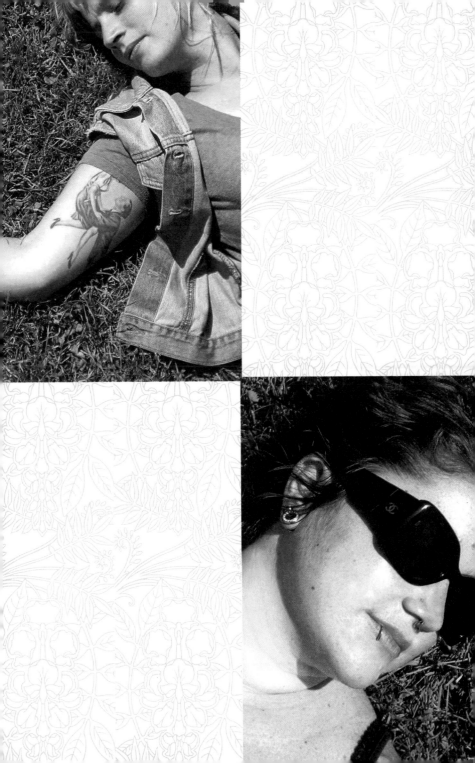

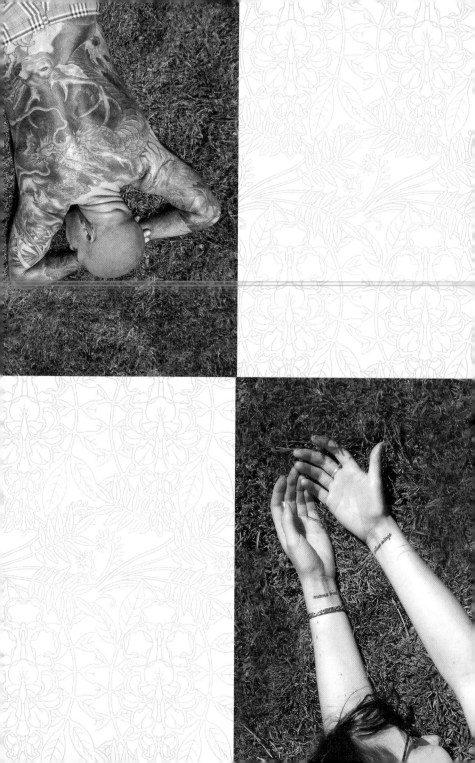

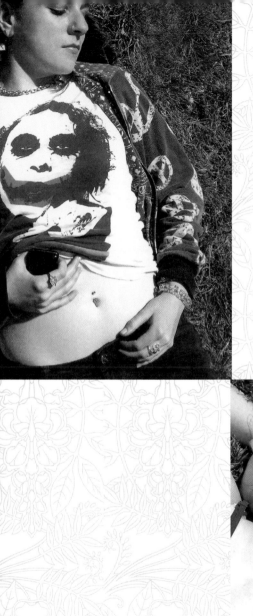
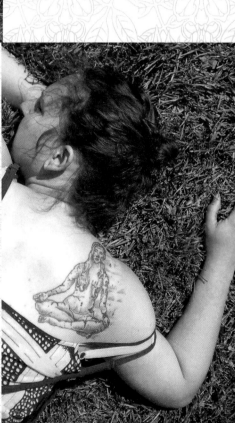

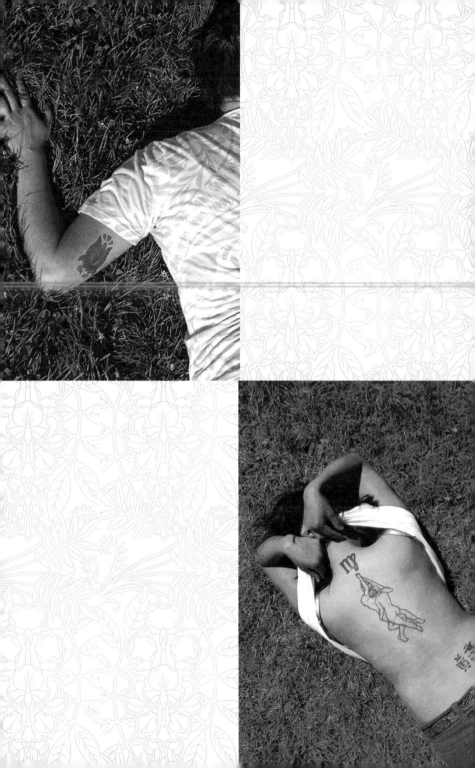

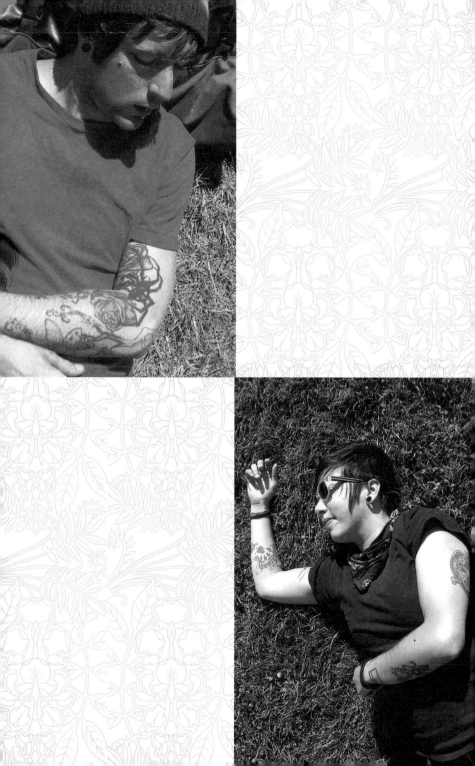

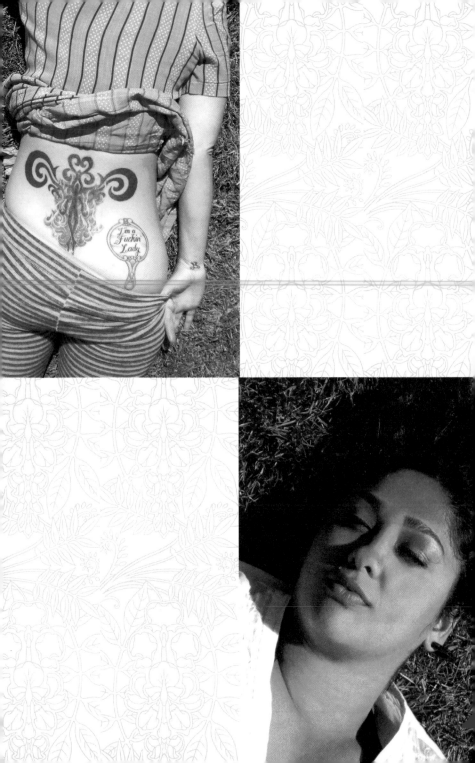

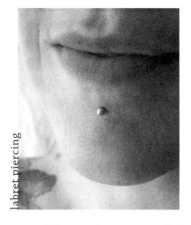

labret piercing

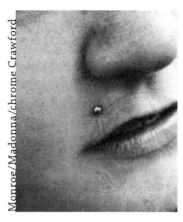

Monroe/Madonna/chrome Crawford

14-gauge labret stud. I recommend that you use the smallest-size back disc possible to reduce the amount of contact it has with your teeth and gums.

MONROE/MADONNA/CHROME CRAWFORD

This piercing has many names because it's meant to simulate the upper-lip beauty marks associated with the famous women noted. It's basically a horizontal upper-lip piercing that's off to either one side or the other. It's adorned with a labret stud, so just a single ball end is visible.

A word of warning about this one, though. This is just my personal opinion, but I've found very few people who can wear this piercing without it just looking like a big zit above their lip. Some facial structures just aren't suited for a beauty mark of any kind, and a piercing protrudes even more than a painted or real mark. A smaller ball end or gem sometimes helps, but if it's too small, it's not very attractive either.

Starter jewelry should be no smaller than 16-gauge, even if you want a really small gem. Ask for the smallest disc back possible to reduce rubbing against teeth and gums.

LIP/SNAKE BITES

A lip piercing is exactly what it sounds like—a piercing through the upper or lower lip, anywhere along the lip line. The difference between the more

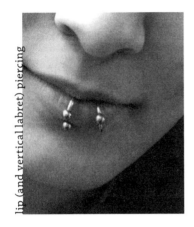

lip (and vertical labret) piercing

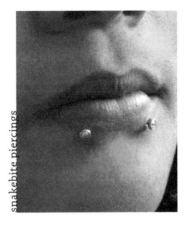

snakebite piercings

generic term and terms like "labrets" and "beauty marks" is that they are usually adorned with a CBR or circular barbell. The bottom lip is usually preferred for this type of piercing, but the upper is also game.

Snake bites are two bottom-lip piercings, one on each side, usually halfway between the center and edge of the lip. I guess it's supposed to simulate fangs; I don't think they look like fangs, but they can look pretty awesome, especially on a full lower lip. Snake bites are usually adorned with CBRs, but some prefer to wear labret studs or circular barbells instead. That's a personal preference, but any starter jewelry should be at least 16-gauge or larger.

> *TIP:* *All body piercings (except genital, of course) are completely unisex. Back in the '80s, there was some connection between left and right ear piercings in men, meaning gay or straight. None of that applies anymore. Most men prefer to pierce both ears now anyway, instead of only one, and that also has absolutely no significance except personal preference. Nostril piercings are typically preferred by women, but plenty of men get them, too; again, left or right makes no difference. So feel free to get whatever you like!*

ᥰ Oral Piercings

TONGUE

I will admit up front that the tongue piercing is my least favorite of all of them. Not because I don't think they look good—I do. My husband and I both had our tongues pierced for a few years. I had a lot of irritation with mine—either my tongue or the roof or the base of my mouth under the tongue was always sore. It seemed to go in a rotation of pain. And we both managed to break a couple of teeth from accidentally biting down on the ball. Four fillings and two root canals later, I have to say that I do not encourage people to get their tongues pierced. But I know that if you really want it, you're going to get it, so I will give you my best advice to help you avoid the problems we had.

First, just in case you're not familiar with the tongue piercing, it's a straight barbell through the tongue. Usually it's a vertical piercing, but I have seen it done horizontally, too. The tongue can be pierced once or multiple times. The most I've seen at once is five, but I'm sure someone out there has managed more.

The tongue can be a tricky muscle to pierce without causing damage, so it requires a knowledgeable piercer to avoid the numerous arteries and veins. No, there isn't a vein in the tongue that can instantly make you die if it's pierced (a common myth), but improperly placed piercings can lead to infection, which can lead to death, as in the case of Daniel Hindle Anderson (Chapter 28).

If you can't stick your tongue out far enough for it to be pierced safely, you may have a restrictive lingual frenulum (see below). Sometimes it can be surgically clipped to improve tongue movement. Talk to your doctor if this is a problem for you.

Starting out with a larger gauge—like a 10-gauge barbell—can help minimize movement that causes fistula discomfort with smaller barbells. It's also important that you switch to a proper-size barbell as soon as your piercing is healed enough; you'll start out with a longer one to accommodate swelling, but wearing a longer barbell than is necessary only increases your odds of accidentally biting down on it.

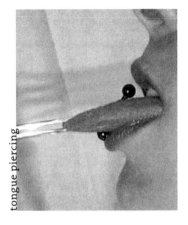

tongue piercing

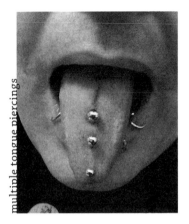

multiple tongue piercings

A lot of piercers will recommend using Listerine mouthwash when caring for a new piercing. I advise strongly against the use of this product. It's too strong and can actually burn your tongue. I still have scar tissue on the surface of my tongue from Listerine burn. Some piercers will say to just dilute the Listerine with water, but since there are alcohol-free products out there, like Biotene, that kill germs just as well, I would steer clear of it altogether.

> *TIP: Don't smoke! Introducing tar and toxins directly into a raw oral piercing is just asking for trouble. And I'm speaking from experience here. I was a smoker when I got my tongue pierced, and I know that's one of the reasons it always felt irritated. Not only that, but smoking slows down the body's ability to heal, which deals a double blow. I'm amazed at how much faster my body heals since I quit smoking. Since it's in your best interest to quit smoking anyway, consider this incentive!*

LINGUAL FRENULUM/TONGUE WEB

The word "frenulum" is used for any thin strand of tissue that connects two body parts in order to serve as a restraint. The more common term is

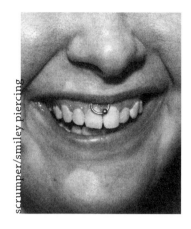
scrumper/smiley piercing

"web," like the webbing on a frog's or duck's feet. We have webbing, too, just in different places. If you look in the mirror and lift your tongue up to the roof of your mouth, you'll see a bit of connective tissue in the center that attaches your tongue to the bottom of your mouth. That's called your lingual frenulum, but most people call it a tongue web. And yes, it can be pierced if it's large enough.

It's usually pierced with a very small CBR—sometimes as small as 18- or 16-gauge. Because of potential irritation due to friction against the bottom of your tongue or the floor of your mouth, smaller jewelry with a smaller bead will be less intrusive. But smaller jewelry also means a greater chance of migration and rejection.

UPPER-LIP FRENULUM (SCRUMPER/SMILEY)

The upper-lip frenulum is the web that connects the upper lip to the gums in the center of your mouth. If you pull your lip up toward your nose, you can see or feel it there. Not everyone's frenulum is big enough for piercing, but your piercer can tell you if yours has ample tissue or not.

It's a very cute piercing and sometimes called a smiley because it's visible to others only when the wearer smiles. The upper lip rides up just enough during a big smile to allow the bottom half of the ring to show. But it's a potentially problematic location because the jewelry—usually a CBR ranging from 18- to 16-gauge—rubs against the teeth and gums with every movement of the upper lip.

LOWER-LIP FRENULUM (FROWNY)

A frowny is the exact opposite of a smiley. It goes through the lower-lip frenulum—the tissue that connects the lower lip to the gums in the center of your mouth. Pull your bottom lip down in a big frown, and you can easily see it in the mirror. It's pierced the same way, uses the same jewelry, and comes with the same risks as a smiley.

> *TIP:* *All piercings are subject to infection, but oral infections pose the greatest risk of all. Since the mouth is so close to the brain, it's a short trip for the infection to travel to the cranium. The mouth also provides the quickest access to the bloodstream, which means an infection could quickly turn into septicemia (blood poisoning). Either of these possible scenarios could lead to death in a very short period of time, even in an otherwise healthy person. See a doctor immediately if you have any pain or swelling in your mouth.*

৶ Body Piercings

NIPPLES

Even though men and women both have nipples, and both can be pierced, the same rules don't necessarily apply to both sexes. Female nipples are attached to breasts, which are sometimes large, and that changes the dynamics of the piercing dramatically. Female nipples also contain developed mammary glands, which some women use to deliver nourishment to their babies, and that presents additional considerations. Last but not least, women are subject to tenderness and swelling of the nipples during certain times of the month. So, simply put, a nipple piercing is a much bigger deal for a woman than it is for a man.

The good news is that despite all this, women can still have their nipples pierced, and it doesn't affect their ability to produce or deliver milk. The bad news is, *because* of all this, nipple piercings can be sore a lot. Sometimes they never feel quite right. Sometimes they just never heal properly. A lot of women give up on them after a year or so because they're tired of always being in pain. But plenty of women also have great success with their nipple piercings. It's up to you if you want to take the chance.

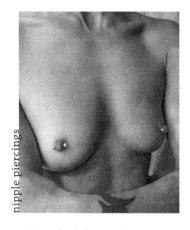

nipple piercings

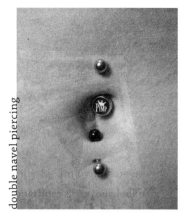

double navel piercing

Men don't have quite as many concerns with nipple piercings, but they do have to have ample tissue to pierce through in the first place. Men are also just as subject to infections and mastitis, which is a painful swelling of breast tissue. Men and women alike share the risk of migration and rejection, since this is essentially a surface piercing.

Nipples can be pierced in a variety of ways—horizontally, vertically, or at any angle, and with a straight barbell, curved barbell, or CBR. I recommend nothing smaller than 14-gauge to discourage migration.

If you have abnormally shaped or inverted nipples, you might still be able to get them pierced, but it will require a consultation with your piercer to determine whether that would be a safe option for you.

Nipple shields are a special adornment made to accent a straight barbell piercing. The shield is held in place with the bar and surrounds the nipple. Because of the weight factor, they should be worn only on healed piercings and only for short periods of time. Otherwise, you risk putting too much stress on the piercing, which could lead to migration.

NAVEL (BELLY BUTTON)

The navel is probably one of the most popular piercings for women, although some men do get it, too. They work best on "innies" (belly buttons that are concave), but sometimes "outies" (belly buttons that stick out) can be pierced as well. Especially with an innie, the navel can be pierced above or below the center—or both. Despite their popularity, they are also *the* most difficult piercings to heal.

If you're going to get a navel piercing, you need to be aware that it could take as much as a year and a half for it to heal. In the meantime, you're likely to deal with a lot of small complications: soreness, redness, bumps, and even minor infections. The navel is not body piercing–friendly and it will fight you all the way. And sometimes you'll lose; a lot of navel piercings reject, and there isn't a thing you can do to prevent it if your body is determined to evict the intruder. But sometimes you'll win and get to keep your piercing. It's a gamble.

The better you take care of your piercing, the better your chances will be of keeping it. It has to be kept clean, dry, and away from tight clothing at all times. Any major stretching or bending is going to cause problems—if you're an athlete, this might not be a good piercing for you. If you've got such a busy life that you barely have time to brush your teeth, this is probably not a good piercing for you. If you're overweight and your navel is often covered by belly rolls (which wouldn't allow the piercing to breathe properly), this probably isn't a good piercing for you. If you're just lazy and don't like things that require a lot of attention, this definitely isn't a good piercing for you.

So, if you've accepted the fact that it's going to take some work, and you're willing to do that, by all means go for it. Just stick to your aftercare regimen and don't give up, even if you face a few small problems along the way.

Large bananabells with dangles and charms are not intended for new piercings; it will only make the healing process more difficult and migration more likely. Start out with a simple 14-gauge curved barbell. I don't think CBRs or circular barbells are a good idea for the navel because they stick out and could get caught on things. Because this piercing is so prone to complications, I would suggest not even trying SSS—just go for niobium or titanium from the get-go.

TIP: Lose the scrubbie! If you've got any surface piercings on your body, I highly recommend that you get rid of the plastic mesh-net body scrubber you have in the shower. They have an uncanny ability to find, snag, and pull on jewelry ends, which can mean instant death to a piercing and a whole lot of pain for you.

ശSurface Piercings

Surface piercings can be very attractive and offer a wide range of placement locations, but they also pose the greatest risk of migration and rejection. It's highly important that your piercer is specifically trained and experienced to perform these piercings, as they require an even greater understanding of the human body than standard body piercings.

NAPE

A nape piercing is named after its anatomical location—the nape of the neck. This is the back of your neck between your head and shoulders, like the scruff on a cat. As far as surface piercings go, it's actually a pretty decent location. The skin is looser there and is usually hospitable to body piercings.

It's usually a horizontal piercing and does well with surface bars or Tygon tubing. Most people prefer flat discs over ball ends, so that they lie flat against the skin and don't get caught on things as easily.

TIP: Out of sight, out of mind? Be extra careful with a piercing you can't see every time you look down or in the mirror. It's easy to forget it's there and accidentally rake across it with a comb or lean against something and put too much pressure on it.

STERNUM (CLEAVAGE)

The sternum is the long narrow bone in the center of your chest, and a vertical piercing along this line is called either a sternum or cleavage piercing. Obviously, men don't have cleavage, but they can still get this piercing if they want to. However, if the muscles are defined and the skin is tight in this area, this wouldn't be a suitable piercing choice.

A lot of piercers will place a curved barbell in the sternum—this is *not* advisable. Sternum piercings are highly disposed toward migration, and the surface tension created by the curved barbell only increases the likelihood of losing the piercing. It should be pierced with a 16- to 12-gauge surface bar or with a biocompatible plastic.

MADISON

This piercing has an interesting history. It was named after Madison Stone, a former adult-film star who now runs her own tattoo shop (Madison Tattoo Shoppe) in Burbank, California. She's a very talented tattoo artist, but she was the first well-known person to wear a horizontal piercing below the collarbone. And so this piercing was named after her.

"My hair would always get tangled up in my necklaces; I went into The Gauntlet and asked if we could just pierce the hollow of my neck so I could hang my charms from it—they looked at me in amazement (probably because they hadn't thought of it yet!), then we marked it out and pierced it. It healed like an absolute dream. I had all sorts of custom charms, crosses, and diamonds made for it. I had no idea it had been named after me until some time later. The flattery of that is inconceivable for most people, to know that you will be immortal because of some simple decision just to make your life easier and express yourself."

—MADISON STONE

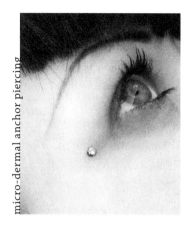

micro-dermal anchor piercing

Because the Madison is located in such a highly visible area and because it's got a high probability of rejecting, you need to consider the scars that will result from losing this piercing. Sometimes the scars fade after a couple of years, but that's a long time to wait if you're not comfortable with scarring.

Even Madison herself no longer wears this piercing and says she probably won't have it repierced. She is now very seriously involved in the martial art Muay Thai and says, "Piercings are not conducive for fighting *at all!*"

A surface bar or biocompatible plastic should be inserted horizontally across the jugular notch—the small depression at the base of the front of the neck. Nothing smaller than 16-gauge should be used; a larger gauge offers a higher success probability.

MICRO-DERMAL ANCHORS

Also sometimes referred to as "single point piercings," micro-dermal anchors are actually a type of surface piercing. The greatest advantage is that instead of having to wear a bar with two visible ends, a single gem or stud can be placed almost anywhere on the body. It stands alone and gives the appearance of simply being stuck on the skin's surface like a sticker, but it's actually quite permanent—more permanent than other body piercings, anyway.

Micro-dermal piercings should be performed with a dermal punch, rather than a needle. It's still a relatively new procedure, and piercers are still learning and experimenting to find better ways to do it, but the ones using a dermal punch are seeing much faster healing times and fewer instances of rejection. There are some exceptions to this rule, and I know some piercers who have tried both and prefer the needle method, but as a general rule a dermal punch seems to be the better option.

The anchor of the jewelry piece is designed in such a way to encourage tissue to grow around it, making it a semipermanent structure underneath the skin. The visible part of the piercing—whether it's a gem, disc, spike, or ball—screws into place, so it can be changed at will.

Although you have a lot more placement options with dermal anchors, that doesn't mean you can put them literally anywhere. They are still prone to migration and rejection just like any surface piercing, and areas of the body where there is a lot of movement seem to encourage piercing evacuation.

The first few weeks, as tissue develops around the anchor to stabilize the piercing, are the most crucial. Any rough movement, bumping, or twisting of the jewel can rip it out or begin the process of rejection. I got two on my chest, side by side—one rejected and the other healed just fine, so then I had one off-center gem and one ugly scar. Sometimes you just never know how these things are going to go.

If you should decide you no longer want your dermal anchor, or if you have to remove it for surgery or some other medical procedure, it's a little more complicated than simply removing a barbell or ring. The skin around the anchor needs to be massaged in order to release the bond between the tissue and the anchor, and then it can be pulled out through the original piercing hole. But it can't just be put back in place once the medical procedure is over—you would more than likely have to let it heal and have it repierced. So, getting this kind of piercing is a much bigger decision than getting any of the others.

TIP: Even though dermal anchors are really just half of a normal piercing, since they have only one entry/exit point, some states have labeled them surgical implants, which can be performed only by a medical professional. You'll have to check first to see if you can legally get this kind of piercing where you live.

✍ Female Genital Piercings

There are several different ways the vulva can be pierced, but not every woman gets to have her choice of what to pierce or how to pierce it. Since female genital anatomy is so varied from one woman to another, it will require a consultation with your piercer to determine what piercings would fit your anatomy best or provide the most pleasure. Jewelry size is largely dependent on your personal anatomy and what you want the piercing to accomplish, so you'll need to consult with your piercer about that as well.

LABIA (INNER AND OUTER)

The labia majora are the soft, fleshy outer "lips" of the vulva. Some women have very thin or small outer labia, while others' are much fuller. Either way, they can be pierced anywhere along the edge of either side.

Outer-labia piercings don't usually provide any additional sensation and are purely for aesthetic value. One popular style is the labial corset, in which both sides are pierced with a row of CBRs and then tied together with ribbon.

Chastity piercings are similar, but actually use the jewelry itself (either long barbells or large CBRs) to hold both sides of the outer labia together. Chastity piercings should not be allowed to interfere with normal body functions or personal hygiene.

Your inner labia may or may not be visible in a resting position, depending on whether they protrude beyond the lines of the outer labia or are much smaller. Either way, most inner labia can be pierced, but the larger, the better. Thanks to our natural defenses, they heal quickly and don't present many complications, as long as you practice good personal hygiene.

TIP: If you're not already well acquainted with your female bits, this is a good time to become so! If you want to get a piercing that enhances your sexuality, you should first understand your own sexual nature and what does or doesn't give you pleasure—both physically and visually. It's also a good idea to know exactly what your anatomy looks like in its healthy state so you can easily identify problems if something should happen to go wrong with your piercing.

Inner-labia piercings may require smaller-gauge CBRs, depending on the amount of accessible tissue. Outer labia can be pierced with a CBR anywhere from 16- to 10-gauge and can then be stretched to even larger gauges if desired. You should avoid sex for at least a week (maybe two) after getting a labial piercing and then use protection and exercise caution for several weeks afterward, until you're sure it's healed.

CLITORIS

When referring to body piercings, a lot of women confuse their clitoris with their clitoral hood. What many women mistakenly refer to as a clitoral piercing is actually a hood piercing. But there are rare cases in which a woman will pierce her actual clitoris.

The clitoris is a very sensitive organ that contains over eight thousand nerve endings. For most of us, it is the key element to sexual arousal and climax. By piercing it, you risk causing irreparable damage to your sexual core. That's a very serious consequence that needs to be considered before attempting this piercing. Your piercer will no doubt give you the same warning.

Not all clitorises are large enough to be pierced anyway, and your piercer will be able to tell you if yours is or not. They are typically pierced horizontally and then embellished with a CBR. No sex for at least two weeks, and then be very careful for at least three months afterward.

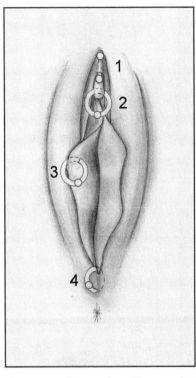

1. vertical hood piercing
2. clitoris piercing
3. inner labia piercing
4. fourchette piercing

CLITORAL HOOD (VERTICAL AND HORIZONTAL)

Probably the number one intimate-piercing choice for women, the clitoral hood piercing provides the most pleasurable stimulation. With the right placement, the jewelry offers gentle friction against the clitoris during both normal movement and sex.

The "right placement" is key, because this piercing will do you little or no good if it's not done just right for you and your body. So you can't just go into a shop and say you want a vertical hood piercing; your piercer needs to examine you first to determine whether a vertical or horizontal hood piercing would be best suited for you.

A deep hood piercing is one that is placed under the skin, behind the clitoral shaft. Remember, your clitoris isn't just that little surface nub you can see; it's much larger than that underneath the surface. Think of it kind of like a bendy straw, bent all the way down, but with two tubes below the bend instead of just one; the short end you would drink from is the part that visibly protrudes. A deep hood piercing has to go far enough

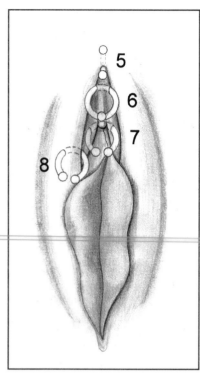

5. Christina piercing
6. horizontal clitoral hood piercing
7. triangle piercing
8. outer labia piercing

into the skin to wrap behind both sides of the bend. If it were to accidentally pierce the back "bend" of the shaft, it could damage those important nerves previously mentioned.

Hood piercings can be adorned with small curved barbells or CBR jewelry. The type of jewelry you wear and its size will also affect how much direct stimulation it provides to the clitoris.

Sex should be avoided for at least a week, and then you need to be gentle for several weeks afterward. If it hurts, don't do it.

TRIANGLE

The triangle is a beautiful and gratifying piercing. But, like most genital piercings, you can get it only if you are anatomically blessed. A triangle is actually a hood piercing, but instead of piercing through the hood above the clitoris, it passes through the hood underneath so that the jewelry stimulates the underside of the clitoris. So for this piercing to be possible, you need to have ample hood tissue and a clitoris that protrudes enough to even have an underside.

A CBR usually provides the best look, comfort, and stimulation for this piercing. Sex should be avoided for at least a week or two, and then extra care should be taken for a minimum of three months.

CHRISTINA

This is actually a surface piercing that goes vertically from the upside-down-V-shaped intersection of the outer labia at the top of the vulva, and exits about an inch higher through the pubic mound (or mons).

Depending on the structure of your mons, this may or may not be a good piercing for you. It tends to be difficult to heal and is prone to twisting or binding with natural body movement, which can be uncomfortable. A flexible biocompatible plastic bar is probably the best jewelry option, so it can be cut to size and move with your body, rather than against it.

Sex doesn't necessarily have to be avoided completely with this piercing, but you and your partner should be extremely careful for at least six months, until it's healed.

FOURCHETTE

If you read the section about oral piercings, then you know what a frenulum is. The fourchette is the triangular frenulum labiorum pudendi at the lower points of the inner labia, just above the perineum.

Not every woman has a fourchette, or some may have been damaged due to intercourse, childbirth, or an episiotomy. If you have one, it can be pierced, but it tends to get in the way during sex, rather than enhance it. Because it's such a fragile flap of skin, it doesn't take much to damage it, so you have to be extra careful with it.

A fourchette is typically pierced with a CBR—larger gauges are better to prevent tearing and rejection. Sex should be avoided for at least two weeks, and then extreme care should be taken for at least three months afterward.

TO THE EXTREME

There are more ways to pierce and modify the female genitals than have been listed here, but I wouldn't recommend most of them. Slight variations on the piercings already discussed here might be okay, but extreme procedures that could ruin your body and sexual enjoyment should be avoided. Always consult with professional piercers and be willing to yield to their recommendations if they're made in your best interests.

ᴄᴏ Male Genital Piercings

There are several piercing options available to men that can enhance sex for themselves or their partner, and others that are more for aesthetic purposes. Depending on what he hopes to gain from piercing his nether regions, at least one of the following should do the trick.

> *TIP: Experienced piercers will not ask—or require—you to have an erection in order to mark or perform any male piercing. Ask your piercer up front if the piercing can be done while you are flaccid; if it can't, find another piercer. On the other hand, piercers completely understand if a man gets an involuntary erection during the procedure, and there is no reason to be embarrassed if that happens—even if your piercer is a guy. It happens!*

PRINCE ALBERT

Even if you have no interest in genital piercings, you've probably at least heard of this one. The Prince Albert (usually just called a P.A.) is by far the most sought-after male piercing. It's a relatively simple piercing and a good healer, but that doesn't mean it doesn't come with its share of caveats.

A standard P.A. enters the frenulum—the underside webbing of the penis that connects the glans (head) to the shaft—and goes into and out the urethra. This piercing is possible on both circumcised and uncircumcised men. A lot of piercers won't pierce directly through the frenulum skin itself, especially on uncircumcised men, so it may need to be placed just slightly to one side.

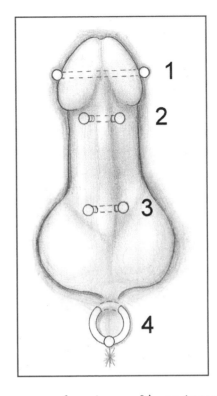

1. ampallang piercing
2. frenum piercing
3. lorum piercing
4. Guiche piercing

After getting a P.A., a man should abstain from sex for at least two weeks. From that point, he should always wear a condom during sex (including oral) for at least three months, even if he is monogamous. This can be frustrating, as the jewelry can cause the condom to tear, which obviously defeats the purpose of wearing one. It's very important that he put the condom on carefully, and it does help to use one that has an extra-large reservoir at the tip.

Most men do report an increase in sensation when wearing a P.A., but not all partners enjoy the feeling of it. So don't assume it's going to enhance your love life—sometimes it does and sometimes it doesn't.

A reverse P.A. is just the opposite of the standard version. Instead of starting at the underside of the shaft, it enters through the top and still exits through the urethra. Both styles are usually adorned with either a CBR or a circular barbell, no less than 12-gauge. P.A. piercings are much more comfortable and risk fewer complications when they accommodate larger-gauge jewelry. Many men will decide to stretch them even larger afterward.

TIP: A Prince Albert piercing doesn't necessarily doom a man to sitting on the toilet to pee for the rest of his life. It might for a while, though, while he "practices" how to handle the change in urinary flow. Some men can actually train their bodies to control the stream while standing, and some decide to opt for a prince's wand, which is a special piece of jewelry made to fit the piercing but that has a removable end to allow for normal urination. Then again, there are also those who just aren't able to get the hang of it or simply prefer to sit—just in case.

FRENUM

Frenum piercings are probably the second most popular for men. A single frenum piercing is a straight barbell through the underside skin of the penile shaft, just below the glans. For an uncircumcised man, this is directly under the frenulum. Even though the frenulum is usually removed during circumcision, the same location can still be pierced on an uncircumcised penis.

Because the frenulum is the most sensitive part of the penis, the jewelry can heighten arousal and pleasure during sex. While both circumcised and uncircumcised men can get a frenum piercing, a frenum ladder—a row of parallel frenum piercings down the underside of the shaft—is an option only for a circumcised penis. Either can get a lorum, however, which is a frenum piercing at the very base of the penis, just above the scrotum. Since frenum piercings penetrate skin only, they're low on the pain scale. They're usually pierced with 14- to 12-gauge straight barbells and are basically surface piercings, so there is a risk of migration and rejection. However, they seem to fare quite well with most men and take only a few weeks to heal. CBRs should be worn in healed frenum piercings only, and caution needs to be taken even then.

Sex should be avoided for about a week, and then a condom should be used every time for at least three months. The more frenum piercings you get at one time, the longer it may take for total healing.

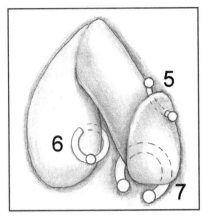

5. dydoe piercing

6. hafada piercing

7. Prince Albert piercing

DYDOE

A dydoe goes through the fibrous material around the outer rim of the glans. The head needs to have a sufficient "cap" shape in relation to the shaft in order to have enough flesh for the piercing to penetrate and hold.

The glans can be pierced anywhere around the rim, parallel to the shaft, and be considered a dydoe. It can hold one, two, or multiple piercings around the circumference of the glans. Dydoes are purported to provide enhanced sexual pleasure to both the man and his partner.

While this piercing is usually best placed on a circumcised penis, uncircumcised men can sometimes adapt to it as well. The major considerations in this case are that the foreskin needs to be loose enough so as not to suffocate the piercing, and extra care needs to be taken to keep the area clean and dry, especially during the initial healing phase.

Dydoes are typically pierced with 14- or 12-gauge curved barbells. Proper jewelry length for a snug fit is important to decrease movement and tension, especially during sex, and to avoid migration or tearing of the skin.

Sex should be avoided for at least two weeks, and then a condom should be worn at all times for at least four months. It can take up to six months or more for this piercing to heal.

AMPALLANG

An ampallang is a horizontal piercing right through the middle of the glans. It is a relatively painful piercing that can seem to take forever and bleed significantly because there's so much fibrous tissue for the needle to penetrate. But once it's healed, it can provide a fair amount of pleasure.

This piercing is an option for both uncircumcised and circumcised men. It's pierced with a straight barbell, usually 14- or 12-gauge. Sex should be avoided for a minimum of two weeks, and then protection should be used for at least six months. This is a slow healer, sometimes taking a full year or more to be considered fully healed.

APADRAVYA

An apadravya is very similar to an ampallang, except that it is a barbell that goes vertically through the glans instead of horizontally. It can be done straight up and down, but it actually fits the anatomy better when pierced at an angle. Theoretically, this might provide more pleasure to a female partner because it could stimulate the G-spot.

The same rules and restrictions that apply to the ampallang apply to this piercing.

TIP: While ampallangs and apadravyas don't have to penetrate the urethra, they can, and there is an advantage to this, as urine is a natural disinfectant that actually helps keep the piercing clean and speeds up healing time. The disadvantage is that it can affect the flow of urine and require the man to sit when he pees. But a lot of men have found ways to adapt and at least be able to use a urinal once they adjust to the change in flow.

FORESKIN

This is obviously one piercing that is pretty much exclusive to uncircumcised men. The foreskin can be pierced anywhere around the perimeter

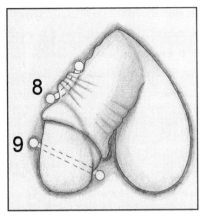

8. foreskin piercing

9. apadravya piercing

that surrounds the glans when the penis is flaccid. It has to be done carefully so that it doesn't tug or rip the foreskin during an erection.

Other than placement issues, foreskin piercings are relatively simple and heal well, although they are subject to migration if the jewelry gauge is too thin. They should be pierced with a minimum 14-gauge curved barbell or CBR. Sex should be avoided for a week, and then a condom should be used until the piercing is healed, which takes anywhere from two to four months.

SCROTUM/HAFADA

The skin of the scrotum can be pierced pretty much anywhere, but there seems to be a general consensus that an official hafada is higher and to one side or the other of the penile shaft. However, the term "hafada" seems to have taken on a more generic definition to mean any piercing of the scrotal skin.

Even though this is technically a surface piercing, it tends to fare better than others due to the elasticity of the skin. And because it is going only through skin and not fibrous tissue, it is relatively low on the pain scale and heals well as long as it's kept clean and dry, which can be a challenge. Piercings along the underside of the scrotum are particularly susceptible to bacteria, due to the dark, moist environment.

Piercing options are diverse, as the scrotum can be pierced horizontally or vertically and with a variety of jewelry styles and gauges, depending on personal preference. It can be pierced once or multiple times in various locations. A vertical row down the center, in line with the penile shaft, is called a scrotal ladder, which can be worn alone or in conjunction with a frenum ladder.

Men who enjoy scrotal stimulation may find this piercing pleasurable during sex, especially if they are wearing heavy or multiple pieces of jewelry. Otherwise, it's more for decorative purposes. As long as direct pulling or squeezing of the scrotum is avoided for a couple of weeks, sex can resume as usual after receiving a scrotal piercing.

A transscrotal piercing that penetrates the entire scrotal sac (usually front to back) is extremely risky and is not advisable, as the consequences could be dire if it's not performed exactly right or an infection develops.

GUICHE (PERINEUM)

The perineum is the stretch of skin between the anus and the base of the scrotum. A surface piercing along this line is called a guiche (pronounced "geesh"), whether it is perpendicular to or in line with the penis.

It's a tricky piercing, as it needs to be given sufficient depth to discourage migration. Larger-gauge jewelry (12-gauge or higher) helps in that regard, too. Healing is also challenging, since it's so close to the anus, which maintains a dark, moist environment, a virtual welcome mat for bacteria. Keeping this piercing clean and dry is very important, especially during the first few weeks.

A guiche piercing won't really interrupt a man's sex life, except for when he receives anal penetration. That should be avoided for at least two weeks, and then extra care should be taken until the piercing is fully healed, which could take a year or longer, depending on how well it's been cared for.

❧In Conclusion

There are more options for male genital piercings—some are simply hybrids of two or more of the piercings already covered here. Some are more risky—even downright dangerous—and I don't encourage trying something that could cause irreparable damage. Since the male ego and self-esteem are closely linked to a man's penis and sexual prowess, attempting a modification that could harm him physically could also result in psychological injury.

There are many more ways in which the body can be decorated or modified, and as long as you have a qualified artist by your side, your options are vast. But there has to be a point where all of us draw the line, because there *is* such a thing as going too far. And sometimes, once you cross that line there's no going back. Self-expression shouldn't be pushed to the point of self-harm or permanent mutilation.

choosing
your piercer

Even though a piercer doesn't have to have the same artistic qualifications as a tattoo artist, it's still very important that you find one that is experienced and qualified. You would think those two words would be synonymous, but not all experienced piercers are qualified and not all qualified piercers are experienced.

Experience is defined as knowledge gained from something that is encountered or repeated over a course of time. In many instances, skill is improved as experience is gained. But if piercers simply repeat the same mistakes over and over, that experience doesn't make them qualified.

One trend sometimes found in the body art industry is a resistance to change. That kind of attitude simply isn't tolerable in an industry that is constantly evolving and improving with those changes. Many practices that were considered the norm ten years ago are now deemed unacceptable. You wouldn't want to get your hair cut by someone who hadn't kept up with the trends in the past decade or more, and you certainly don't want to be pierced by someone who hasn't followed improvements in safety measures.

On the flip side, being qualified is a more desirable trait to find in a piercer, but it isn't a stand-alone requirement. Piercers may have been trained properly, learned all the latest methods, and follow sanitation procedures to the letter, but that doesn't give them experience. If they've only been piercing for a short period of time, then they haven't had the opportunity to encounter all of the ups and downs that go along with the art. The more piercings artists do, and the more problems they have to overcome, the more experience they add to their qualified status. What you want is a piercer so comfortable with what they do that they could practically perform it in their sleep.

When you combine experience with qualification, you have the recipe for an excellent piercing experience.

༒ Piercing Specific

All piercers are not both qualified and experienced in all piercing forms. Some of them may be especially proficient in performing surface piercings, while others are better at dealing with sensitive cartilage. What you need to look for is a piercer that meets the requirements of the specific type of piercing you are looking to get.

If you desire a piercing that is newly invented or you have come up with an idea of your own that you want to try out, you need to acknowledge the fact that you are not going to get the benefit of experience and that things may go wrong. In this case, at least look for a piercer who is qualified and also confident when it comes to trying new things. Some of them really enjoy a challenge, while others may be intimidated by the idea.

New piercing styles are constantly being introduced, but some piercers want to wait them out and learn from others' mistakes before trying them out themselves. I know of one shop piercer who will try out a new style on all of his coworkers at the shop first, documenting and learning from each person and how their bodies react, before he will attempt it on a paying customer. I think this is a great practice, but not many piercers do this. Don't assume that just because a certain piercing is "all the rage," your piercer has already had a chance to perform it.

∽ When in Doubt, Walk Away

The "golden rule" of body art is that if you're in doubt, don't. If you don't feel 100 percent confident in your piercer's abilities, don't just sit there and let them pierce you because you don't want to offend them. This is your body, your health, and ultimately your life; your piercer is not your best friend, they are a business partner. And you have every right to make a business decision to walk away.

the piercing studio

Most tattoo studios also offer piercing services, but that's not always the case. When searching for a shop, you can usually begin by looking for tattoo studios. But in some rare cases, there are piercing-only shops, especially in areas where tattoos are banned. The reason most shops offer both services is that they usually depend on both trades to sustain the business. Tattoos bring in the most money, but piercings can keep a shop going during the slower times when there isn't as much demand for ink. Shops that offer only one service or the other usually find themselves struggling.

Whatever kind of studio you decide to visit, you need to examine it on two different levels. First, you need to inspect the studio as a whole: Is it clean? Is the staff friendly? Are they certified and/or insured in accordance with your local laws? Do they practice Standard Precautions?

In order to get answers to the above questions, poke around a bit. Dust, cobwebs, a dirty bathroom, and dirty or overly cluttered workstations are not good signs that anyone working there is too concerned with cleanliness. An unfriendly and unhelpful staff gives the impression that they are not concerned with the needs of the client. Not being up to date with insurance and required certification is a huge red flag.

Ask for a tour of the place—if they're happy to show you around, especially if they point out their sterilization area, that's a good indication that they have nothing to hide and want you to feel comfortable. If they don't show you the sterilization area, ask to see it. If they hesitate or seem disgruntled by the request, leave.

ᕲᑐ The Piercer

Once you've determined that the studio is acceptable, you need to then examine the piercer(s) and their practices. The first thing you'll want to do is just talk to them. A short consultation between the two of you to discuss the piercing you want will tell you whether you feel confident in their abilities and feel comfortable with them as a person.

With some piercings, it may be necessary for you to have an actual physical examination of the body part to determine if you are anatomically adequate. For example, if you want a scrumper, your piercer needs to look inside your lip to make sure your frenulum is large enough to support the jewelry. If you want a clitoral hood, your piercer needs to see first if you are better suited for a horizontal or vertical piercing.

Sometimes you can go straight from the consultation to the piercing room if your piercer is available and you are ready. But don't feel that you have to do it that way. You can also make an appointment for a later date if you wish.

Once you're in the piercing station, remember that you still need to be alert. It's easy to get swept up in the experience and forget that you're still supposed to be inspecting the situation to protect your safety.

> *TIP: Any doors and/or windows of the piercing room should be closed automatically or at your request. If you feel uncomfortable with the idea that you're alone in a closed*

room with your piercer, you can also opt for the door to be left open, unless it's for an intimate piercing. But to be honest, if you feel vulnerable in a closed room with the piercer, then something is telling you not to trust them. If that's the case, you shouldn't be there in the first place.

They should wear gloves anytime they touch your skin and change gloves after coming in contact with anything besides your skin or the materials used to pierce you. All equipment—needles, jewelry, receiving tubes, clamps, etc.—should be presterilized or new and disposable.

The entire area surrounding the piercing location should be cleaned thoroughly. Whether they use clamps or pierce freehand, they should take time marking and lining up the piercing path to make sure it enters and exits the skin properly. Even the pen for marking the area to be pierced (skin scribe) shouldn't come in direct contact with your skin unless they plan to throw it away after using it on you. My piercer touches the tip of a toothpick to the tip of the scribe and then uses the toothpick to mark my skin. It may seem like a small detail, but it's a detail I appreciate because it shows the lengths she is willing to go for her clients.

If your piercer has already failed to follow any of these most basic practices, get out before it's too late. Simply excuse yourself—tell them you've had a change of mind—and leave.

If everything is kosher, though, this is when you'll actually get the piercing. And this is when a lot of us begin to panic. The next couple of chapters will help you prepare for and deal with the most difficult sixty seconds you'll spend in the piercing shop.

what to bring
with you

Before you can get pierced, there will be some paperwork you will need to fill out. That paperwork requires a signature—either your own, if you're of legal age, or that of a parent if your state allows them to sign for you.

If you're old enough to sign for yourself, you'll need identification. A state ID or driver's license are the only forms of ID accepted in most shops. (Other government-issued identification forms, such as a birth certificate, may be accepted, but it's best to call the shop first and ask.) If you're underage but can have a parent sign for you, then obviously you need to bring that parent, and *they* will be required to have legal identification. Sometimes a shop will even require that the adult show proof of guardianship or custody, especially if their last name is different from yours, to prove you have permission for the piercing from the person responsible for you.

The other thing you'll obviously need is money. Many shops only accept cash; some will take credit cards, but very few accept checks. If you're not sure what forms of payment your shop will accept, call first and ask. Tip money for your artist is always best as cash; that way, you are sure that the tip goes to the right person.

Since a piercing is over so quickly, you really don't need to bring things to distract you. In fact, you really shouldn't bring things that will disrupt the communication between you and your piercer. It's important that you are both talking and listening through the procedure to make sure everything is going right. You'll need to check the markings and approve the lineup, and then you'll need to let them know if anything feels terribly wrong during the piercing itself. Afterward you'll have to inspect the finished piercing and get instructions on how to care for it, so reading or listening to music really isn't helpful or respectful. You can bring these things in case you have wait time before you are seen, but put them away once you're in the piercing booth.

You can, however, bring a friend with you for support. Unless the piercing booth is extremely small and there just isn't room for another body, your piercer should have no objection to your having a friend with you. Having a friend to hold your hand or make you laugh can make the procedure much less intimidating and even seem to pass more quickly.

It's always nice to ask first, but you can usually also bring a camera or video camera and have a friend document the piercing. Don't try to take pictures yourself if you don't have a friend with you, though, as it would only make it more difficult for you to relax and harder for your piercer to do their job. Also, respect your piercer if they prefer not to be included in the photos and/or video.

> *TIP: Dressing appropriately before certain piercings is also helpful. Clothing that restricts access to the area of your body that is getting pierced can make you feel uncomfortable or necessitate the removal of clothing. For example, wearing a skirt or dress is much easier when getting a genital piercing, since the skirt can simply be pulled up, instead of your having to completely remove a pair of pants.*

what to expect

This chapter will break down the process of getting a piercing, step by step, from the moment you enter the shop until you leave with your new piercing. Keep in mind that all piercers are different and may have their own ways of doing things. As long as they are keeping you clean and safe, variations in actual piercing methods are fine.

✄ Step 1: Walk-in or Appointment

Because piercings are relatively quick procedures, most shops welcome walk-ins, meaning they don't require that you make an appointment beforehand. However, if you have a tight schedule and can't afford to wait until the piercer is free, it's best to go ahead and make an appointment anyway. Either way, the first thing you have to do is walk into the shop.

Hopefully you've already followed the advice in the previous chapters, and you know the shop is clean and safe. You've also brought along everything you need to fill out the paperwork, which is the next step.

TIP: Since some shops have more than one piercer, you might prefer one over the other, and that's fine. If you want to be pierced by a specific artist, make sure you know what days and times they work, or you might end up making another trip.

ॐ Step 2: Paperwork

Don't be scared; just walk up to the counter or the first employee who acknowledges you and tell them you would like to get a piercing. Let them know if you've made an appointment and which artist you would like to see, if you have a preference. Once they know what kind of piercing you want, they will ask for your ID and hand you a paper to fill out.

The paper will ask for basic information like your name, address, birth date, etc. It will probably include a disclaimer, *which you should take the time to read,* and then ask some more specific health questions. Being dishonest about any health conditions could put you in danger, so it's very important that you answer the questions honestly!

Then you sign and date the bottom of the page, and that paper is usually then attached to a photocopy of your ID. Now you're ready for your piercing.

ॐ Step 3: The Piercing Room

Most piercers have a private room, not an open booth. If they use a booth, that is fine as long as there's a curtain or some other way to protect the client's privacy.

Most of them also utilize a long, padded table—like a massage bench. Some states require that all stations have running water, so there may be a sink. There will probably be a shelf with containers of different items, such as cotton balls, cotton swabs, oral antiseptic, rubbing alcohol, gloves, and other tools of the trade. However your piercer's room is set up, it should be clean and inviting.

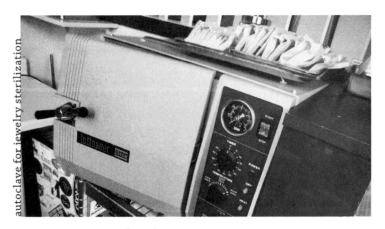

autoclave for jewelry sterilization

Step 4: Dot Marks the Spot

After inviting you to sit down, your piercer will clean your skin where you'll be getting pierced. Depending on what kind of piercing you're getting, your artist may use rubbing alcohol, Green Soap, oral antiseptic, or a mild cleanser for the genital region.

Once the area is clean, the piercing entry and exit points will be marked with a dot. Then your piercer will allow you to look at the dots in the mirror and approve the placement. This is the time to speak up if it seems off in any way. Once you've given the okay on the dots, it's time for the needle.

Step 5: Pop Goes the Needle

This is where many of us—even seasoned pros at getting pierced—feel a little anxious. You may get butterflies in your stomach or feel a little queasy. That's perfectly normal. But it's because of this reaction that your piercer will probably have you lie down, no matter what kind of piercing you're getting. I remember being really confused when I was asked to lie down for an eyebrow piercing, but it's just a precaution. Sometimes the endorphins that kick in as a result of anxiety can make us feel a little faint. If you're already on your back, there's no chance of falling down if that happens.

If your piercer prefers to use clamps, this is when he/she will use

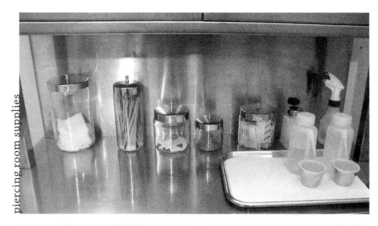

piercing room supplies

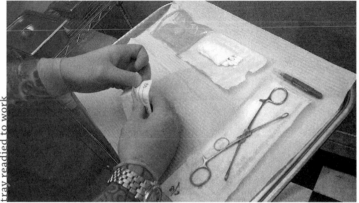

tray readied to work

them to pinch the skin and hold it firmly in place. Some piercers prefer to do it freehand—either way is just personal preference. I actually like it when my piercer uses clamps, because the squeezing of the skin kind of numbs it just a bit, making the piercing less painful.

To keep you as calm as possible and make the piercing as painless as possible, your piercer will ask you to take a few slow, deep breaths. You'll feel just the point of the needle against your skin as you breathe, and then your piercer will follow a nice, strong exhale with the insertion of the needle tip. Depending on how much tissue the needle has to penetrate, it may go all the way through on that exhale. If not, it's probably very close to being done anyway. A couple more breaths usually do the trick. I've never had a piercing take more than sixty seconds from start to finish, but that can feel like a very long sixty seconds when a needle is being pushed through your flesh.

If you're getting a cartilage or surface piercing, you may hear a slight *pop* as the needle breaks through the skin. That's perfectly normal. As far as pain goes, I have found that breaking through the skin on each side of the fistula is the most painful part, while the needle traveling through flesh in between those two points is more annoying than painful. My worst reaction to the most painful piercing I've ever gotten—my industrial— was gritting my teeth really hard for a few seconds.

TIP: Some piercings may cause your eyes to water, but that doesn't necessarily mean that you're crying! It's just a natural physiological reaction, just like if you were to yawn or pluck your eyebrow hairs. No need to feel silly if you shed a tear or two—it's not the same as breaking down, and it can happen to anyone.

Step 6: Inserting the Jewelry

Once the needle is all the way through, you can take a deep breath and relax. Your piercer will probably let go for a moment while they get the jewelry ready. Some of them will use a receiving tube, which enters the piercing first and helps feed the jewelry through the hole. Or they may simply use the jewelry itself to follow the end of the needle. Either way, the jewelry base—whether it's a barbell, a CBR, or something else—will be inserted and then closed. Sometimes the closing of the jewelry is another sharp pinch of pain, but it's over and done very quickly!

Step 7: Listen Up!

Most piercings don't bleed much, but there may be a drop or two that needs to be wiped away. If you have a bleeder, though, don't worry. Your piercer will clean you up the best they can and give you instructions on how to handle it if it continues to bleed at home. My dermal anchors took about an hour to stop bleeding. Some male genital piercings have been known to drip for a week or so. This is the point where you really need to pay attention to your piercer so that you know what is or isn't considered normal for your piercing.

While they are cleaning you up, they will also give you verbal aftercare instructions. Again, pay attention. If you don't follow the aftercare properly, you could screw up your new piercing. This is also the time to ask any questions you might have about aftercare, the healing process, the jewelry, or anything else you might want to know about your piercing. Try not to drag the conversation on for a long time (so your piercer can get to the next client), but don't be afraid to speak up. Their reputation and livelihood depends on your having a successful piercing experience, so they are more than happy to help you make that possible.

∽ Step 8: Before You Go

Once you leave the room, it's back to the front of the shop to pay for your piercing. If you haven't already tipped your piercer, you can do that now. You will also be handed a set of written aftercare instructions to serve as a reminder. Sometimes they will even give you the products they recommend for aftercare. My piercer gives all of her clients a bottle of Satin antimicrobial cleanser, a small plastic baggie of sea salt, and a cup to use for soaking, all of which are included in the price of the piercing. I think this is an excellent way to ensure that clients use the right aftercare products, but not all shops do this. At the very least, they may sell the products they recommend. If not, then make sure you know exactly what you need to look for when you go to the store.

Once you've gotten your instructions and paid for your piercing, you're all set. Take care of your new baby and don't hesitate to call your piercer if you have any questions or problems. Free upkeep advice is part of the service.

healing and aftercare

Once you walk out the door of the shop, your piercing becomes your responsibility. It's up to you to take care of it and keep it healthy so that it can heal. That doesn't mean your piercer won't help you, but it's still your job to call them if you need them. Your piercer can't be blamed if you drop the ball and end up with a serious problem.

If you didn't walk out of the shop with the aftercare products you need, and you don't already have them at home, then the first thing you need to do is go to the store to get your supplies. Waiting two or three days to go to the store is going to start you off on the wrong foot. The first few days are the most critical.

If you're not sure what kind of aftercare products to get, you can either ask your piercer or follow my recommendations. I always suggest that you default to your piercer's advice first; since you trusted them to pierce you in the first place, you should also trust them to know what products are best to take care of the piercing. However, I feel that it doesn't hurt to get a second opinion or have a few more options to choose from in case one thing doesn't work for you or if your piercer isn't available.

᧥Dos and Don'ts of Aftercare

I'm actually going to start with the don'ts because a lot of people get bad advice from boutique piercers, friends, family members, etc., and end up causing themselves a lot of unnecessary grief. The wrong products can cause major healing problems, and when it comes to piercings, there are a lot of bad products that are routinely recommended by well-meaning but ignorant folks.

ALCOHOL

Rubbing alcohol, isopropyl alcohol, drinking alcohol . . . it doesn't matter which—alcohol is bad for any fresh wound and certainly shouldn't be used to clean a piercing. All you manage to do is irritate the wound and kill some of the surrounding tissue, which actually delays healing rather than helping it. It's best to avoid any product that describes itself as being antiseptic, which is a pretty good indication that it's going to be damaging to raw tissue.

HYDROGEN PEROXIDE

It's one of the first things we used to grab for any wound to kill germs, and actually the last one you should be turning to. Similar to alcohol, hydrogen peroxide actually damages healthy cells and invites infection by delaying the healing process. Save the H_2O_2 for household cleaning.

EAR CARE SOLUTION

The little bottles of liquid sold at most piercing boutiques contain a mixture of hydrogen peroxide and a bunch of other stuff that does more harm than good. It's just one of the reasons people experience so many infections when pierced at these places.

GLY-OXIDE

This is a hydrogen peroxide–based product that some will try to use for oral piercings. Hydrogen peroxide isn't any healthier inside your mouth than it is outside your body.

OINTMENTS

Anything thick, gooey, sticky, or creamy should be kept away from your piercing. All ointments manage to do is clog pores and slow healing. And no, antibacterial ointments won't cure an infected piercing; there are other solutions for that problem.

HARSH SOAPS

Strong antibacterial soaps and medicine-enhanced cleansers are too strong and will only irritate in the wound and dry out your skin.

LISTERINE

This is a highly recommended product, even by some experienced piercers, but it has been found to cause more problems than it solves. Even diluted, it's too strong and ineffective at keeping germs at bay.

Now that you know what *not* to use, the next step is to learn what products are safe and will help the healing process.

PROVON OR SATIN ANTIMICROBIAL CLEANSERS

Both of these products are approved for use in the medical industry and have proven themselves to be strong enough to kill germs but mild enough not to harm healthy cells. They are both available in different areas, so your location may determine which of these products you'll be able to find; both are equally respected.

> *TIP: There's still a heavy debate going on as to whether or not antibacterial and antimicrobial soaps are really necessary to wash away germs. It seems that most regular soaps, and even just plain water under healthy conditions, are just as effective in removing bacteria from skin surfaces. But the studies that have reached this conclusion were not dealing with wounds— only surface skin. They also don't change the fact that many*

"regular" soaps contain perfumes and other ingredients that would definitely be unwelcome in a fresh piercing. Provon and Satin cleansers are, if nothing else, devoid of harmful agents and mild enough to use daily without drying the skin or killing healthy tissue. These cleansers have a clear record of aiding in the healing of body piercings for many years.

NON-IODIZED SEA SALT

When you think salt, you probably hear the phrase "pouring salt on a wound" in the back of your mind. While it's true that dousing a cut with table salt would cause pain and burning, sea salt actually has a very soothing effect on raw tissue when mixed with water and used properly. (See my instructions for sea salt soaks in the aftercare section.) It also has the ability to draw out pus and heal the beginning stages of an infection.

SALINE SOLUTION

A bottle of plain saline solution—not the kind made for cleaning contact lenses, but a pure saline wash—is a good substitute for sea salt. It also makes a good travel companion; throw it in your purse, and you can clean your piercing anywhere, anytime.

BIOTENE

This mouthwash, which does not contain alcohol, has been found much more effective than Listerine and at the same time is great for overall oral and dental health. It's a win-win.

TEA TREE OIL

This is a natural oil with antiseptic *qualities* (not the same as a harsh or chemical antiseptic) that soothes piercing irritation and can heal up minor infections. Some people find the aroma of tea tree oil offensive, while others find it inviting. Never use tea tree oil at full strength; dilute it with water (one part oil, one part water) first.

EMU OIL

This is a natural oil that is extracted from the meat of the flightless bird. Pure emu oil has a wonderful ability to soften and moisturize the skin without clogging pores. It can be difficult to find, especially pure in quality, and is rather expensive.

∾ "Iffy" Options

There are other products out there that have been used for healing piercings, and while I don't necessarily advise *against* them, I would call them iffy. You can try them and if they work for you, great. If they don't work or—even worse—cause you problems, don't use them.

At the top of my iffy list is Bactine spray. Some people can use it and it works great, while others find that it dries their piercings out or irritates them. The APP (Association of Professional Piercers) advises against it, and with good reason. It does contain some chemical ingredients—including nonoxynol 9 (huh?)—as well as an antiseptic agent and fragrance. But, as I highly recommend this product to ease the burn of a new tattoo, I don't have any prejudice against it; it seems to have a pretty mild effect on most people. If you find it works for you, then by all means go ahead. I wouldn't use it *every* time, but maybe occasionally or just during that first day or two to relieve the burning sensation.

The other products I would consider iffy are the ones that have been created and marketed specifically for the piercing industry, such as H2Ocean, X-pression (by Tattoo Goo), Love My Piercing, and other similar aftercare lines. There is nothing *wrong* with these products, per se, but I wouldn't consider them necessary when there are many other less expensive and more readily available products to choose from. If you prefer one of these specially made products and it works for you, then that's fine. Some people swear by them, while others feel they're a waste of money. Personally, I stick to simple methods and products that offer additional uses after my piercing is healed.

৶ Skin Piercing Aftercare Instructions

The first day you get your piercing, you don't need to do a whole lot to it, except avoid exposing it to anything harmful. It was already pierced under clean conditions, and it's good to just leave it alone and allow it to calm down a bit. If it's still actively bleeding, you can blot it with a tissue as needed. I don't recommend using cotton balls or swabs because tiny cotton fibers can get caught in the piercing and lead to problems.

Make sure you sleep on clean sheets, and I recommend changing your sheets and pillowcases every two days during the healing process.

The next morning is when you'll need to wash your piercing for the first time. You may see a dry crust around the piercing hole(s); this is just dried-up lymph that the piercing will secrete for the first few days. This is perfectly normal, and the "crusties" are easily washed away with warm water and a little cleanser. Using just your hand, splash warm water around the piercing or hold a cup of warm water up against it for about ten seconds, to soften the crusties. Then put a drop of cleanser on the tip of your finger and gently work it around the piercing site and the jewelry. A few more splashes of water—taking care to remove all cleanser and any remaining crusties—will soothe your piercing, as well as clean it.

Once you have thoroughly cleaned your piercing, gently blot it dry with a clean washcloth or towel. If you have an additional product you'd like to use, such as tea tree or emu oil, put a drop on the piercing and allow it to dry on its own. That's all you need to do to clean your piercing, but once a day you should also do a sea salt soak.

৶ Sea Salt Soaks

Take a small pinch, about an eighth of a teaspoon, of sea salt in a small cup (I like to use the little two-ounce condiment cups) and mix it with about two ounces of hot—as hot as you can stand it—water. If you have hard or sulfur water, you should use distilled water for the best results.

Hold the little cup of salt water against your piercing if possible—allowing a seal to form between your skin and the cup rim—and hold it there for five to ten minutes. If you can't hold the cup against your piercing, then soak some gauze with the sea salt solution and place it over your piercing. It will cool off quickly this way, so you might want to keep rewetting the gauze every couple of minutes. Using this indirect method, you should treat your piercing for no less than ten minutes.

Once your sea salt soak is finished, gently rinse away any salt residue with warm water and pat dry with a clean towel.

> *TIP: You can make a sea salt solution and put it in a squirt bottle to carry with you and use anytime you need to refresh your piercing. It won't be hot, which is the most effective way to do a sea salt soak, but it will do in a pinch and is better than nothing.*

✑ Oral Piercing Aftercare Instructions

Piercings inside the mouth require different care than those on the body. Since we use our mouths for so many things—talking, eating, drinking, smoking, kissing, etc.—it's easy to see why oral piercings are so vulnerable from the start. The good news, though, is that our mouths are very good at fighting germs naturally, and all you really need to do is keep your mouth healthy so it can do its job. So, healing an oral piercing is not about treating the piercing specifically, but about oral and dental hygiene.

The first thing you should do is buy a new toothbrush. Starting fresh will ensure that you're not brushing your teeth with something already laden with bacteria. It should have soft bristles, too, so it's not too harsh on your gums and palette. Then, brush your teeth at least twice a day, which is no different from a normal oral-health routine.

If you normally use harsh alcohol- or peroxide-based mouthwash, don't—not for at least a couple of months. I recommend using Biotene or something similar that effectively kills germs without damaging the healthy cells trying to repair your piercing. Don't use any tooth-whitening products during this time, either.

Another effective oral rinse is the sea salt solution mentioned previously. This solution is perfectly safe for your mouth, is able to kill germs, draws out pus and dead cells, and is inexpensive to make. It may not taste great, but you can rinse out with fresh water afterward. I even keep a bottle of premade sea salt solution in the shower and rinse while I'm bathing.

For the first couple of weeks, your mouth is going to be sore, and you have to do everything very delicately. Chew carefully, talk slowly, and don't drink beer. It's best to avoid all alcohol, but the yeast in beer is even harsher on your piercing than straight alcohol. And if at all possible, *don't smoke*. Smoking invites all kinds of nasty toxins into your mouth that are not conducive to healing. On top of that, smoking in general causes your body to have to work harder to heal anything and just isn't good for you.

You can't avoid eating and drinking, but everything else should be put on hold for at least the first two weeks. But if you must engage in other activities, you have to take extra care of yourself. It's important to rinse your mouth out *every* time you introduce anything into it. After you eat, after you drink, after you smoke, or after making out, you must wash your mouth out before bacteria can make itself at home in your piercing. They do make flavored condoms and dental dams, which you should use for the first few weeks if you're going to perform oral sex.

Keeping your mouth healthy will, in turn, keep your piercing healthy. Because of the mouth's close proximity to the brain and direct access to the blood system, you should see a doctor immediately if you think you might have an infection.

✺ Things to Avoid

During the first few weeks of healing your new piercing, there are a few things you need to stay away from.

Swimming pools, ponds, lakes, and oceans are off-limits. They either harbor bacteria, contain harmful chemicals, or both. So don't get a piercing just before a vacation on the beach!

The use of sprays, oils, lotions, creams, gels, makeup, and anything else you're not using to care for your piercing should be kept away from it for a few weeks. If you need to apply hairspray or perfume, remember that they spray outward and cover a lot more area than you can see. Cover your piercing up before you apply anything that could harm it.

৩ Expected Healing Times

The time it takes to heal a piercing is as individual as people themselves. It can be greatly affected by personal health, diet, activity, environment, and adherence to aftercare instructions. So identical piercings on two different people could take very different lengths of time to heal. It should also be mentioned that there is a difference between healed and *healed*. A piercing can be healed in that it isn't sore anymore and feels fine, but that doesn't mean all the tissue on the inside has completely repaired itself. Complete healing of most piercings can easily take a year or more. That being said, I can at least give you some estimated healing times.

Soft-tissue piercings, like earlobes, eyebrows, and vertical labrets, are the easiest to heal, usually taking only four to six weeks. Cartilage and septum piercings, barring any serious problems, usually take eight to twelve weeks to heal. Surface piercings are more complex and can take as long as six months to heal. Oral piercings heal rather quickly, in as little as six weeks, but are easily prone to setbacks. Combination oral/ skin piercings are slower to heal, usually taking eight to twelve weeks at the least. Nipple piercings on men usually heal faster than they do for women—usually in about three months—while female nipples may take twice that amount of time. Navel piercings tend to be highly problematic and can take anywhere between six and twelve months to heal, sometimes even longer. Most genital piercings heal up in about six months, although some can heal quicker if they don't go through a lot of flesh. Adherence to sexual restrictions and hygiene is especially important to encourage healing of genital piercings.

gauging up: how to enlarge your piercing

If you want to increase the size of your piercing hole so that you can wear plugs, flesh tunnels, large-gauge claws, etc., it's called gauging up. Gauging up can be done a few different ways, and it's important that you learn how to do it safely. Gauging up too much, too fast, or the wrong way can cause irreparable tissue damage, collapsed cartilage, or severe scarring.

✺ Capered Stretching

The most popular way to gauge up is to gradually stretch a piercing from one size to the next until you finally reach your desired gauge. It's a very slow method and requires patience. A taper is the tool used to accomplish this. It's a thin bar of metal that is small and pointed on one end and gradually increases in girth, by either one or two gauges, up the length of the bar, which is usually around four to six inches long. A lubricant, such as K-Y jelly, is applied to the tip of the taper, which is then inserted into the piercing hole. Very slowly, as the wider sections of the bar pass through the hole, it gently stretches it to the larger size. A new piece of jewelry in the new gauge size follows the end of the taper, and then you've successfully completed your first stretch.

A tapered stretch can be performed *only* on soft tissue (never cartilage) and should not be attempted on a piercing that is not completely healed. The stretch should never be more than one or two gauges at a time, depending on the size you start with. Going from a 16-gauge to a 14- isn't much of a stretch, but an 8- to a 6-gauge would be too much at once, since the gauges increase exponentially as the numbers decrease.

Once you have stretched, your piercing will go through a healing process similar to the one you experienced when you first got pierced. It's important to allow it to fully heal—yes, again—before you attempt another stretch. Gauging up several sizes could take years if done properly.

Another way you can do a tapered stretch is by using metal talons or claws that are tapered. Just the process of wearing them and slowly moving the jewelry farther up over time will allow for a nice, safe stretch without any trauma.

✆ Weighted Stretching

There are special weights made to be hung from piercing rings that gently tug on the piercing, encouraging it to stretch. It's not the best method, though, because it could tug too hard and end up damaging tissue anyway. The biggest problem with using weights, though, is that the piercing hole isn't stretched evenly on all sides of the fistula as it is with tapering. Instead, the bottom of the piercing takes the brunt of the weight and sags, while the top and sides may stretch unevenly or not at all. The likelihood of the skin's ever being able to return to its original shape is also very slim when it's stretched in this manner.

✆ Dermal Punch

A dermal punch is a tool used for removing a section of flesh, rather than pushing it aside or stretching it. It's actually the same tool used to take tissue samples for a biopsy, and it comes in a variety of gauge sizes. The

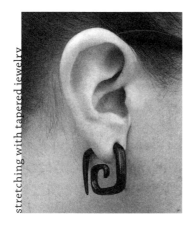
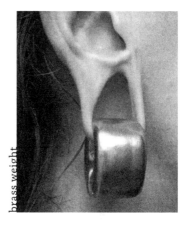

stretching with tapered jewelry

brass weight

circular-shaped blade at the end cuts out a matching circular hole in the skin, like a cookie cutter cuts out a shape of dough.

It sounds more traumatic than it is. The dermal punch isn't forced through the skin like a hole punch through paper. Usually, a little pressure is applied as the punch is rotated back and forth so that it gently slices the tissue until it works its way through. That's not to say it isn't painful, though, because it is. And there's a good deal of bleeding associated with removing an entire chunk of skin. But it is the only way to gauge up a cartilage piercing safely. You should never try to stretch cartilage; it doesn't have any elasticity and can be badly damaged if you try to force it to expand.

A dermal punch can also be used on soft tissue and even surface skin for dermal anchors. The main disadvantage of this method is that there's no going back. You can't regrow the flesh that was removed, so you will always have the hole. That's actually the case with a lot of stretched piercings, but not all.

> *TIP: There are some new dermal punches showing up on the market that offer different geometric shapes, such as hearts and stars. Since these shapes can't be rotated like the round dermal punch, pressure is the only way the blade*

can penetrate the skin. That's not necessarily a bad thing, but make sure you've got a gentle and sympathetic piercer if you're worried about pain. Experience is also a must, since the products are relatively new and you don't want them playing guinea pig with you.

∽ Will It Shrink Back?

If you decide you no longer want a stretched hole, is there any hope of its shrinking back to its original size and shape? Well, there are several conditions that may or may not make that possible.

- How long has it been stretched? If you've had your lobes stretched for ten years, there's a very good chance that they're settled the way they are and aren't going to shrink back if you remove the jewelry.
- How big were they stretched? Everyone has a "point of no return" where the tissue just isn't willing to reform once it crosses that point. Unfortunately, there's no way to really know where that line is drawn for each of us, so all you can do is try and hope for the best.
- Was it stretched too fast, and did the tissue develop scar tissue? If too much damage to the skin has been done, it's not likely to return to its original state.
- How old are you? Youth does have its advantages. The younger you are, the quicker your skin bounces back from these things and the better your odds are of the hole shrinking back.

Since there's no way to predict whether your piercing will revert if you change your mind about stretching, it might be best to be really sure about it before you gauge up.

troubleshooting

Even if you and your piercer do everything right, it's always possible for something to go wrong. You're placing a foreign object into your body, and sometimes you just can't predict how your body is going to react. The only thing you can really do is try to identify the problem, treat it, and hope for the best.

∾ Piercing Just Won't Heal— Red, Swollen, Itchy, Rashlike, Flaky Skin

All of the above symptoms are usually a sign that you're having an allergic reaction. If that's the case, you need to know what your body is reacting to before you can do something to fix the problem.

If you have metal hypersensitivity, there is a good chance you might have a reaction to your jewelry if it contains nickel. Costume jewelry, stainless steel, and even sterling silver can contain enough nickel to cause problems in people who are allergic to it. Signs of nickel sensitivity include itchy red patches, flaky scales, discolored skin, or small watery blisters in the area surrounding the piercing. The major complaint I hear is that the piercing just won't heal, even after months of care.

You can go to a doctor and have a skin patch test done to confirm a nickel allergy, but you can also replace the jewelry with a higher-grade metal, such as niobium or titanium, and see if the symptoms improve. Don't just remove the jewelry, though; wash the piercing thoroughly and replace it with something else so the hole doesn't close up. Any professional piercer can do this for you so that you don't injure your piercing.

Since nickel accumulates in the body over time, you could develop a sudden allergy to it at any point during your life. So even if you don't have this problem yet, it's really best to avoid nickel as much as possible anyway.

> *TIP:* Even some foods contain nickel, such as cocoa, legumes, broccoli, dried fruits, and canned produce. The more nickel you introduce into your body now, the more likely you become to develop hypersensitivity to it later.

An itchy, pink, or red rash around the piercing that is not caused by nickel could indicate an allergy to the aftercare products you're using. Since there's such a wide range of products available, it's difficult for me to know what yours might contain that is causing you problems. What I would recommend in this case is to simply stop using your aftercare products— change to a different but very mild cleanser and nothing else for two to three days, and see if the rash subsides. If not, let your piercer take a look at it. It's much easier to diagnose a problem when you can actually see it.

౬ Dry, Flaky, Itchy Skin Around Piercing Site

These symptoms usually indicate irritation rather than an allergic reaction. It's milder and the itching comes from the skin being dry, not because of a rash. This usually means that whatever you're using on your piercing is too harsh or you're simply doing it too often. Even soothing sea salt soaks can dry and irritate your skin if you do them more than once a day or use too much salt. Some cleansers are harsher than others or may contain chemicals that irritate your skin. Stop using whatever you have been and try something new. You can call your piercer for recommendations, but make sure to stay away from alcohol- or hydrogen peroxide–based products.

ᘒ Swollen, Red, Dot, or Seeping Pus; Fever; or a General Ill Feeling

Although an allergic reaction can certainly be annoying, an infection is much more serious. But infections sometimes start out looking like an allergy—a few little bumps or itchy, swollen, raised skin. While the symptoms may seem similar at first, something very different is going on beneath the surface.

An infection happens when the body is invaded by harmful foreign cells. Bacterial pathogens are the largest concern when talking about body piercings. There are many different strains of bacterial infections, some of them minor and others life-threatening. It's important that you take *any* infection very seriously, because even a minor one can turn dangerous in a short period of time.

Zeke Wheeler of Missouri, age fifteen at the time, decided to pierce his own lip one day with a household needle. His immune system was already compromised because he had bronchitis, but he was taking antibiotics for that. His mom caught him in the bathroom and put a stop to it, but the damage had already been done. Within just a few days, Zeke had been to the ER two times with complaints of fever, joint and muscle weakness, and severe cold sweats. The sweating was so bad it necessitated the changing of his bedsheets several times a day.

Each time Zeke was dismissed, the doctors assuring his mother that he probably just had the flu. His symptoms continued to get worse, and then his mom noticed that he had red spots on his palms and feet, and in his mouth. After the third emergency room visit, he was finally admitted into the hospital, where he ended up staying for six weeks. The infection that riddled his body damaged his heart and required multiple surgeries of his joints and five blood transfusions. It nearly killed him. Even now, he has a heart murmur and faces another surgery in ten to twenty years because of the damage the endocarditis did to his heart valve, which will eventually need to be repaired.

> *"Who would have told him this was dangerous? It's not something you're educated about. Honestly, I never, never would have thought that because he pierced his lip, the result would be this."*
> **—JILL HANLIN, ZEKE WHEELER'S MOM**

Signs of localized infection are as follows: tenderness, redness, swelling, skin that is hot to the touch, and the presence of pus that is white, yellow, or green in one small area surrounding the piercing and nowhere else. This is when you want to get control of the infection or see a doctor before it gets out of hand. In a matter of days, a localized infection can progress to cellulitis (infection of the connective tissue, which spreads quickly), septicemia (blood poisoning), MRSA (antibiotic resistant strain of staph infection), and many other complications—such as the endocarditis and emboli that Zeke Wheeler suffered—that could eventually shut down vital organs or destroy brain cells. *Infections should not be taken lightly.*

Signs of systemic infection are more flulike: red streaks across the skin, swollen lymph nodes, fever, chills, shaking, diarrhea, and vomiting. If you have any of these symptoms, even if you think they couldn't possibly be related to a recent piercing, go to the emergency room immediately and have it checked out. You may not have time to "wait and see what happens."

⁓The Dreaded Bump

Any piercing can fall victim to "the bump," but cartilage piercings usually give people the most problems. Ear cartilage and nostril piercings almost always grow some kind of ugly bump around the piercing hole; it can happen on the inside or the outside, but unfortunately we're not usually lucky enough to have it grow somewhere hidden. No, instead we get to walk around with a hideous zit-looking thing that not only stands out like a sore thumb but hurts like one, too!

The "bump" can have a variety of characteristics and be caused by different things. Some are more like a blister and can be filled with clear liquid or blood, while some are just a buildup of extra tissue. Sometimes they're just a swelling of the thinner surface layer of the skin, while others originate deeper beneath the dermis and raise a larger area of skin, like a small cyst.

Possible causes of these annoying piercing bumps are metal allergies, sebaceous cysts, hypertrophic scarring, boils, or follicular cysts. Each one may respond to one, all, or none of the following treatments, but it won't hurt to give them a shot; they are often successful.

TIP: If you successfully treat a bump but it reoccurs after a few weeks or months, then you may need to see a doctor. You could have an overactive gland, and sometimes removal of the entire gland is necessary to discourage regrowth.

JEWELRY CHANGE

If you have a metal allergy, then it could be your jewelry that's creating the problem. Change out your jewelry to something made with titanium and see if the problem clears up on its own.

HOT COMPRESSES

A hot compress held against a piercing that is full of fluid or blood will help draw out the fluids and can soothe it by releasing pressure. But it won't prevent it from returning, so once it has ruptured, you should begin the next treatment.

SEA SALT SOAKS

Make a salt solution twice as strong as the mixture I recommended in the aftercare chapter for normal healing. Let it soak as long as you can, at least twice a day. If that doesn't work, you can try some of the next ideas.

CHAMOMILE TEA BAGS

Brew a cup of chamomile tea and then place the hot tea bag against your piercing. Keep it there until it turns cold; do this at least twice a day for two or three days.

ASPIRIN PASTE

Sometimes a more stubborn bump might be dissolved with a paste made of pure aspirin and water. Apply the paste to the bump, leave it there for about half an hour, and then rinse off. Try this a couple times a day for a few days. Be careful to apply this paste only to the bump itself, because it could eat away at healthy tissue, too.

TEA TREE OIL

Tea tree oil is rather strong in its pure state, and it's usually not recommended to use it full strength on the skin. But if you've got a stubborn bump that just won't go away, go ahead and apply 100 percent pure tea tree oil to the bump only—don't get it on any surrounding skin—and leave it there until the next time you wash, at which time you can apply some more oil. Keep doing this until, hopefully, the bump is gone!

> *TIP:* *While these bumps are not initially a sign of infection, once a boil or cyst ruptures, it is at risk of becoming infected or spreading bacteria to other parts of your body. It's very important to keep it clean until the bump is gone or at least resealed.*

ઝ Large Growths (Keloids)

Not to be confused with hypertrophic scars, keloids are similar in nature but a much bigger problem. Hypertrophic scarring is a small amount of additional tissue that grows around a site of injury. It's usually not very big and, as noted in the previous section, it can usually be removed with a little care.

Keloids, on the other hand, are the product of overactive scarring on a much larger level. Your body just doesn't know when to stop mending itself after an injury and builds more and more scar tissue until it usually expands way beyond the boundaries of the initial wound.

For some reason, keloids seem to be more prolific in people with darker skin pigment, but anyone can get them. As if getting a keloid isn't bad enough, most doctors don't recommend trying to remove them. Since injury is what causes them in the first place, trying to cut them off surgically could make the problem worse. You can always ask your doctor for their recommendation, though, because every case is different.

ઝ Piercing Has Moved—Jewelry Is Visible Through the Skin

When a piercing moves from its original location, it's called migration. It generally happens with surface piercings—ones with both entry and exit points on the same plain. Friction, tension, or injury to the piercing can begin the process of migration. It might move just a fraction of an inch and settle into its new location without too much problem. If it continues to migrate, to the point where the piercing is always sore and then you notice that there is very little skin supporting the jewelry anymore, that's called rejection.

Rejection is actually a natural response to "foreign invaders" and is usually a good thing. Once your cells determine that the jewelry is too large and too durable to destroy like they would a small splinter, they seek to evict it instead. The cells begin to build up scar tissue behind the jewelry to force it out through the skin's surface. If you notice this happening, there really isn't anything you can do to stop the process. It's best to remove the jewelry before it actually does push all the way through, which will result in even more scarring.

The good news is, if you've had a piercing reject, you can try again once it's healed up. I usually suggest you give it a few months first. You will have some scar tissue from the original piercing, so getting it redone may hurt a bit more than the first time, but the presence of that scar tissue in front of the piercing can actually discourage rejection a second time.

⁓ Jewelry Has Sunk Down into the Skin

This one's a doozy because it can lead to a very serious problem. It's called embedment, and if your jewelry becomes completely embedded inside your skin, nothing but surgical removal will get it out. Fortunately, you usually get plenty of warning that your piercing is heading in that direction, so it can be corrected.

The first thing you'll usually notice is a small indent in your skin where the end of the jewelry rests. The end of the bar—whether it's a ball or a spike or a flat disc—will nestle down into the indent. The pressure from that nestling will enlarge the piercing hole and eventually become large enough for the jewelry to slide down inside it. For a while, you'll be able to force it back out, but it will only work its way back down into the hole. Eventually, it slips down far enough to allow tissue to close over it, which completely envelops the jewelry. Not fun.

As soon as you start noticing those first signs of embedment, go to your piercer. It's usually easy enough to stop with a longer bar, larger gauge, or larger ball end. Letting it progress, hoping it will "fix itself," will only lead to a bigger problem.

⁓ Piercing Has a Funky Smell

Sometimes this is a normal part of the healing process, but if it's really bad or persistent, then it could be a couple of different things, the first being low-grade jewelry. If your jewelry contains any metal alloys that are not biocompatible, you might be having a reaction to it, which can cause your piercing to smell funny.

The other possibility is that the smell is coming from dead skin cells mixed with sebum, lymph, and other bodily fluids. Those things are supposed to be washed away with each cleaning, but sometimes buildup can be particularly stubborn. Carefully clean the area, using a saline "pressure wash" if necessary. Make sure you're rinsing thoroughly when you wash around your piercing so soap residue isn't getting built up around the site.

If the smell is accompanied by redness, itching, or soreness, it could be a yeast or fungal infection, in which case you need to see your doctor.

piercing FAQs

∾ How Do You Blow Your Nose with a Nose Piercing?

Very carefully! Seriously, for the first few weeks after getting your nostril or septum pierced, blowing your nose is a delicate process. You don't want to damage the piercing, so you have to be careful not to squeeze or wipe your nose too hard. But the additional germs that are introduced to the piercing by bringing mucus to the front need to be cleaned away after blowing your nose, which I recommend you use a saline wash for. It needs to be rinsed out and wiped dry—preferably with a clean, lint-free cloth or gauze—after sneezing or blowing. The once simple process of blowing your nose becomes a more complicated practice, at least for a few weeks, but it's worth it in the end. Once your piercing is completely healed, you can blow your nose in a more "normal" fashion and usually won't even notice that the piercing is there.

Can Two Tongue Piercings Get Tangled Up with Each Other While Kissing?

It's rare, but yes, it can happen, especially if the barbells are different in size or length, which gives them more opportunity to get hung up on each other. But I don't know if I've ever heard of this becoming a situation that required intervention from a third party to pull the entwined kissers apart. Usually it's just a little catch that is easily fixed with normal movement. More times than not, you just hear a lot of clicking sounds when the barbells come in contact with each other, which could definitely ruin the moment if it makes you laugh!

Why Do Piercings Have to Be Removed for X-rays?

Getting an x-ray with piercings in won't harm you, but it can mess up the x-ray results. Body jewelry shows up as dark black shadows in the shape of your jewelry, and since the picture needs to show everything from one side to the other of your three-dimensional body, that black shadow could block out something very important anywhere in that particular line of sight.

Why Do Piercings Have to Be Removed for MRIs?

MRI stands for "magnetic resonance imaging." The way it works is by using a very powerful magnetic field that is strong enough to attract and realign the hydrogen protons in your body. A magnet that strong would also pull very hard on any ferrous (magnetic iron) metal in your body, including body piercings. The pulling of jewelry out and away from your body at this extremity could tear your skin. Some types of nonmagnetic metals have also been affected on occasion, so it's simply best to remove any instance of metal from your body. Ask your doctor first if they're okay with your wearing nonmetallic jewelry for the interim during your MRI scan.

✋ What Should I Do If I Accidentally Swallow My Jewelry?

Swallowing jewelry from an oral piercing happens more often than you'd think. Sometimes it's the whole thing and sometimes it's just one piece. Either way, most jewelry can pass through the digestive system without any problems. You may or may not actually see it when it exits the body, but it should pass within a few days. If you experience any pain or discomfort in your chest, stomach, abdomen, or bowels, though, it could indicate that the jewelry has become lodged somewhere or possibly even punctured something. Go to the doctor immediately, before it threatens your health.

✋ Can Body Jewelry Attract Lightning?

There actually was a news story in which a teen boy was struck by lightning and doctors blamed his tongue ring, which was blown out of his mouth during the strike, and his tongue was left with a big, black hole. The Canada Safety Council, however, says that while metal and electronic items on the person being struck by lightning do cause more contact damage, they don't actually attract the lightning in the first place. The American television show *MythBusters* did a segment to test the likelihood of body piercings attracting lightning. Their conclusion was that it would take a piece of jewelry as big as a doorknob to directly attract a bolt of lightning, but they admitted that the pierced dummy did attract more indirect lightning strikes. I'd say the only way to have a clear answer to this one would be to know the mind of a lightning bolt. Sometimes freaky things just happen.

✋ Does Body Jewelry Set Off Metal Detectors?

Most security metal detectors, such as those at airports and government buildings, are designed to detect dangerous items: guns, knives, bombs, etc. Since the settings on the machines are adjustable, they're usually set high enough to ignore small metal objects that pose no danger, especially if they're made of nonferrous metal. I've been through airport and event metal detectors with over a dozen piercings and have yet to set one off. A few forgotten coins last year, though, sent me back through the stupid thing twice. Go figure.

✧ Can a Woman Still Breastfeed If She Has Pierced Nipples?

Nipple piercings do not affect a woman's ability to breastfeed. She should, however, make sure that her piercings are well healed, showing no signs of irritation or infection that could be passed on to the baby. The jewelry should be removed and the nipple cleaned before nursing, to remove any possible bacteria inside the piercing itself. Leaving the jewelry in could cause difficulty with latching on or even choke the child if the jewelry happened to fall off.

✧ How Do I Remove My Jewelry?

Body jewelry is a little tricky to open and close, but once you get the hang of it, it's not a big deal. If it's a CBR, then it's the tension on each side of the circle that holds the ball in place. There's a special tool called ring-opening pliers that you can get to pry the sides of the ring apart, which releases the ball, or you can use traditional pliers wrapped with electrical tape. (The electrical tape cushions the pliers so the metal doesn't scratch the jewelry. Scratches invite bacteria growth.) As you carefully pry the ring open just a bit, be prepared to catch the ball when it falls out. To close it back up, you need to push the sides back together close enough that the remaining open space is just a bit smaller than the ball. Then you push the ball into the opening and allow it to "pop" back in place. You can also get ring-closing pliers to help with the job, or just use your hands if the gauge isn't too thick.

If it's a barbell, the first thing you need to know is whether one end screws on and off or both. If it's only one, you don't want to waste your time trying to unscrew something that is permanently attached. You can take a close look at both ends of the jewelry and see if one looks different from the other, or just try to think back to when you got it pierced. Which side of your barbell was your piercer holding when they screwed the ball in the first time? If you really can't remember, just try getting one end off and remember the rule—lefty loosey, righty tighty. If all else fails, you can always go to any professional piercer and ask them to help you remove or change out your jewelry.

> *NOTE: Do* not *remove your jewelry if your piercing is red, swollen, or oozing any fluids. This can cause the piercing to close and the bacteria/infection to be trapped inside the skin. With nowhere else to go, the infection could travel to other areas of the body and make you very ill.*

permanent cosmetics

Cosmetic tattoos are a wonderful option for people of all ages, and there's a wide variety of reasons for getting them done. They're often called permanent cosmetics because of the stigma associated with tattoos, but that is exactly what they are. Pigments are inserted underneath the skin to create an illusion, rather than a picture, but that is the only major difference.

There's a variety of reasons to get permanent cosmetics, which is why the clientele base is so varied. While an older woman may want tattooed eyebrows to simulate natural hair that has been lost, a younger woman may want her lips done to create a fuller appearance.

There are three basic ways in which cosmetic tattoos are usually applied. A traditional coil machine, like the ones used for regular tattoos, is probably the most popular method used. Another way is with a rotary machine, which looks like an electric pen but works like a tattoo machine, only at a slower pace and with less power. The final way is by manual insertion with a hand tool that has a small group of needles at the end.

Manual insertion may sound barbaric or primitive, but it actually allows the artist much more control over the way the color is deposited, since they're working on such a small, sensitive area to begin with. It's less traumatic to the client's skin, which shortens healing time, and there's no buzzing machine sounds or vibrating against your skull. It's no slower than any other method and just as permanent. The most trusted manual-insertion system is called SofTap. I don't want to sound like a commercial, and I promise I'm not getting any kickbacks from the company, but I really do believe that this is the best option when it comes to cosmetic-tattoo techniques. So I sought out the help of one of my friends, Jane Adler, who is one of the most renowned and respected permanent-cosmetics artists in the country—and she also happens to be a SofTap technician.

I had the pleasure of spending the day watching and learning about the process from Jane at her shop—Facial Art by Jane in Phoenix, Arizona. There's so much to this art form that it could be a book unto itself, but I'm going to just cover the basics so you get the gist of what it's all about.

✪ What Can and Can't Be Done

There are several different options when it comes to permanent cosmetics. Eyebrows, eyeliner, lip liner, and full lips are the most commonly chosen applications. But there are some misconceptions in regard to these procedures because many women think that if they get these things done, they'll never have to apply makeup again. Permanent cosmetics are not a replacement for daily makeup. Eyeliner will make your eyes look more youthful and alert, but not "made up." Even lip color is meant to enhance your lips, not make them look like they already have lipstick on them. Most of the time, even after getting permanent cosmetics, you'll still want to apply regular makeup over it for a complete look.

Most women wear makeup on their eyebrows to fill in bald spots or add more shape and dimension to them. That is one problem that can be corrected with permanent cosmetics. Once your brows have been filled in, you shouldn't need to resort to the pen or powder anymore.

Areola restoration—also called micropigmentation—can make a huge difference in the life of a woman who has lost her natural nipples due to a mastectomy or an accident. Permanent cosmetics can be used to create realistic-looking areolas with or without the presence of actual nipple tissue.

Sometimes small patches of skin that have lost pigment can be corrected, but dark birthmarks and large areas of discoloration from skin diseases such as vitiligo are beyond the scope of what permanent cosmetics can accomplish.

↶ Is It Really Permanent?

Any time color is inserted into the dermal layers of the skin, it is permanent; this goes for standard tattoos as well as cosmetic. It can't be washed or scrubbed off, and the particles of pigment remain underneath the skin unless they are removed with laser treatments.

That being said, "permanent" doesn't mean those colored particles can't fade. In fact, for most of us, there is a very good chance that they *will* fade over time. This is especially true with permanent cosmetics for a few reasons. One is that your face is the highest point on your body and is exposed to the greatest amount of sun. The sun can fade pigment under your skin just like it fades the paint on a house.

Cosmetic tattoos are also more vulnerable because they don't have as much to protect them from the elements. We don't usually wear clothing on our faces, and we usually neglect daily sunscreen use. Not only that, but the skin protecting the pigment is much thinner on the lips and eyes than it is on the rest of your body.

Finally, we tend to do more to our faces in the way of chemical peels, wrinkle reducers, and other skin enhancements that wear away at the protective skin and sometimes penetrate deeply enough to break down some of the pigment.

So, even though cosmetic tattoos are permanent in most respects, they still may have to be touched up from time to time. How often varies from one person to the next; you could need a touch-up once a year, and then again, you might be able to go ten years before you need one.

✣ An Eye for Color

One of the reasons Jane is so good at what she does is because her gift for understanding color is probably the most crucial part of creating pleasant-looking cosmetic tattoos. Without proper knowledge of how the pigments work with the skin and what it takes to create the right effect, the results could be disastrous. Since many clients seek out permanent cosmetics because they're already self-conscious about a certain trait they aren't happy with, the last thing they need is for someone to make them look and feel worse. Working on someone's face is an incredible responsibility, and you want to find an artist who takes that responsibility very seriously.

Permanent-cosmetics colors are chosen to *complement* your natural skin tone, hair, and eyes, not to match your eyes or what you happen to be wearing that day. Unlike the regular makeup you may put on each morning to decorate your face, permanent cosmetics are meant to enhance.

> *TIP:* Since all color choices are selected to harmonize with your skin tone and natural coloring, it won't affect the look of properly applied permanent makeup if you decide to change your hair color.

✣ Preparation Before the Procedure

One of the first things you'll do before getting any permanent cosmetics is have a consultation with the artist. During that consult, your reasons for wanting the procedure, your color preferences, and your medical history will all be discussed. Then your artist will recommend what colors would suit you best for the procedure you want to have done. Colors don't look the same once they've been tattooed underneath the skin, so part of your artist's job is to be able to predict the outcome when your skin has healed over the pigment color, which is not something every cosmetic-tattoo artist is good at.

The pigments themselves are available from many different companies, just like tattoo inks; some of them are good and others are not. Permanent cosmetic pigments are not regulated by the FDA (Food and Drug Administration), so the companies making them are not required to follow any specific safety rules. Jane, who chooses the best products she can find, stays away from anything that contains FD&C or D&C dyes, which have been linked to allergic reactions. She also prefers to use iron oxides, as they have been used for many years and have proven themselves to be safe.

> *"I met Jane a few years ago to have my eyebrows filled in. I plucked them too much in high school and messed them up. They just don't grow back right after that and drawing them on looked fake, so I decided to give permanent cosmetics a try. I'm a fifty-two-year-old woman who had never seen a tattoo shop and I was thinking in my mind that it might be a little sleazy, but I was surprised. I've since turned my sister on to it as well, and we both got our eyeliner done. I would trust Jane with anything."*
>
> **—THE BABE WITH THE BEAUTIFUL EYEBROWS,**
> **PHOENIX, ARIZONA**

There are a few things you'll need to do in advance to prepare for a cosmetic tattoo. For about a week prior, stay out of the sun and don't get any chemical peels or harsh facials if you're getting anything done on your face. If you're getting eyeliner, you'll want to be prepared with new contact lenses if you wear them and new mascara; you don't want to risk using something that has bacteria on it. If you're having your lips tattooed, you might want to get a prescription for an oral antiviral medication from your doctor or dentist, since fever blisters are very common after lip procedures. You also might want to arrange for a ride home if you're getting eyeliner, especially if your eyes are very sensitive to the light.

For a few days before the procedure, you will also want to avoid tweezing, waxing, tinting, lash perms, hair depilatories, and bleaching creams anywhere near where you'll be getting tattooed. You will also need to stay away from alcohol and any blood-thinning products. If you typically need to take antibiotics before a dental procedure, you'll want to get some before this as well.

If you take prescription medications, some of them can interfere with successful results. If you use Retin-A or Renova, Jane recommends that you stop applying it for a full thirty days before getting any cosmetic tattoo. You need to be off Accutane for an entire year to ensure it's completely out of your system. That may be a long time to wait, but that's better than wasting money on a tattoo that could damage your skin.

TIP: For your own safety, you should check with your doctor before getting any elective cosmetic tattoo if you take prescription medications or have an illness that may be of concern. It's important to cover these things with your tattooer as well, as they may want a letter of clearance from your physician stating that it's safe for you to proceed.

Tools of the Trade

When an artist uses the SofTap system, the tools for creating cosmetic tattoos are very simple. A sterile setup is the key, which includes all disposal items: alcohol prep pads, gloves, gauze, cotton swabs, a SofTap handle and the necessary needle configuration, a palette to dip into for pigments, and a topical numbing ointment. Other items may be used for various procedures to help hold the skin taut or to protect other areas of the body while working, but that is the basic setup. Everything is manual, so there are no cords or plugs, which makes it much easier for your artist to work gently and consistently, even in sensitive areas.

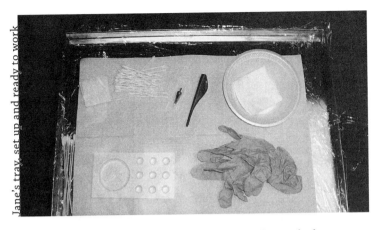

Jane's tray, set up and ready to work

"I feel that the hand and coil machine methods are the best. You can buy a fancy digital machine for an obscene amount of money, but it does not create a better artist. I stand firm that it is the artist behind any method that creates success."

—JANE ADLER

ᕱ Getting Started

Planning out the procedure can sometimes be a slow process, especially if you have an artist whose attention to detail is like Jane's, which is a good thing! Jane takes great care to find exactly the right shade of pigment and to predraw the lines she wants to follow when preparing lips or eyebrows. She will have her clients turn their heads in all different directions and make lots of funny faces while she takes note of how their features react to movement to get just the right look.

Once she's ready, Jane settles her client down on a nice, comfy facial bed—facial not included. Then she cleans the area to be tattooed with an alcohol prep pad or antibacterial soap. Now, this is when most artists would apply a topical numbing cream to the area being tattooed, but Jane works a little differently in this respect. She will prenumb eyes before working on them, but brows and lips require a defined design to look just right, and applying ointment would rub away the lines she draws beforehand. So what she does is follow the outline she made for herself first, and then apply the topical anesthetic, which actually works faster and better once the skin has been broken. She has tried many different methods over the years and has found this to be the best way, and gets no complaints from her clients. They scab less and heal faster when the smallest amount of ointments possible— both before and after the procedure—is used.

๛ The Sound of Success

So, once the client is ready, Jane dips the needles into the pigment and starts working. This hand-poke method is very similar to traditional Japanese *tebori* in concept. It requires an experienced hand to rhythmically *tap-tap-tap* the pigment into the skin evenly and efficiently. The more you work the skin, the more you damage it, so it's important to lay the color as solidly as possible with each tap. And while there aren't any buzzing machines to hear with this method of color insertion, it does make a very distinct sound. Each time the needles are pulled up from the skin, there is a funny, staticlike sucking sound, very similar to the sound of pulling two pieces of Velcro apart. This is the sound of success, because the absence of it would mean the needles didn't penetrate far enough under the skin and the color won't hold.

Does it hurt? Yes and no. I mean, sure, it's uncomfortable, but that doesn't mean it's unbearable. A lot of women have said that tweezing their eyebrows hurts more than getting them tattooed. If anything genuinely *hurts,* your artist might be doing something wrong. Especially if you've been numbed up beforehand, there should be very little discomfort, and if you haven't, the pain shouldn't be any worse than annoying little pricks against your skin.

> "The first few seconds hurt a bit, but Jane tells you exactly what she's doing through every step. It felt kind of hot, like a sunburn. I actually expected it to hurt and be red like when getting a regular tattoo, but it was very different."
> —MARISOL D.

✑ Healing and Aftercare

Jane recommends very limited aftercare; her motto is "less is best." She does send each client home with a tiny container of salve, a few cotton swabs, and instructions on how to care for their new cosmetic tattoo.

Not all tattoos will be complete after the initial session. To produce full color, some areas—especially lips and areolas—could need two or three sessions. To help retain the most color, limit your sun exposure as much as possible for at least a week or more before getting any tattoo procedure.

After any of these treatments, you may not want to use your best bed linens for a while because residue from the pigment and ointment will stick to your pillowcase when you sleep.

EYELINER

It's very normal for your eyes to be swollen and tender for a few days after this procedure. You may even wake up in the morning with your eyes stuck closed, but they can be gently pried open with a wet cotton swab. Itching is also a normal reaction.

Ointment should be applied twice a day, and Jane recommends a "wipe on, wipe off" method to remove any unnecessary product.

Contacts and eye makeup should not be worn for at least three days. Hot tubs, pools, and sun exposure should be avoided until the area is healed; wear sunglasses whenever possible. Any creams or sprays should also be kept away from the eye area during the healing process. Don't rub or pick at the area.

The most common health risk with this procedure is a case of conjunctivitis, which can range in severity from mild irritation to acute infection. It's easily treatable but highly contagious, so get to the doctor as soon as you can.

EYEBROWS

Minor swelling, redness, itching, and a darkening of the eyebrows are all normal parts of the healing process. Jane explains that the darkening is caused by the oxidation of the pigment that is still on the surface, but after about a month, once all the dead skin cells and surface pigment are sloughed away, the true brow color comes through. She likens it to how our hair appears darker when it's wet and even darker still when product is applied; you don't get the sense of the true color until it's dry.

Ointment should be applied twice a day for a week using the "wipe on, wipe off" method. It's important that you don't allow your brows to become dry or crusted.

Don't get any makeup on your eyebrows for at least three days. Avoid swimming, hot tubs, sun exposure, and direct water pressure for at least a week.

"The first time I looked in the mirror after having my eyebrows done, I wanted to cry! I wasn't prepared for the dramatic change, even though Jane warned me they would become thinner and lighter over time. I was still not consoled because I had to go to work the next day. It has now been about seven weeks since I had it done, and they are still in the process of lightening up. My best advice to anyone who is contemplating this procedure is to know going in that the end result will not be what you see when you first look in the mirror. Now I have no regrets about having permanent brows. It is such a relief to not have to draw them on, and when you get out of the shower or the pool they are still there. I have gotten a lot of compliments on them."

—MARSHA P.

LIPS

Lip tattooing is more complex than other permanent-cosmetics procedures, and it requires the most commitment from the client in order to heal successfully. Lips are particularly resistant to pigment saturation, usually requiring at least two or three treatments, and the healing time is consider-

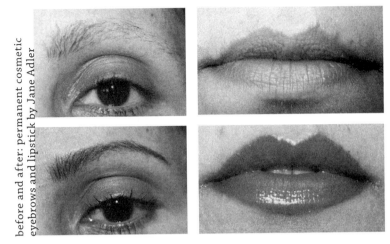

before and after: permanent cosmetic eyebrows and lipstick by Jane Adler

ably slower than that of eyes or brows. Because we use our mouths for so many different things, the list of restrictions during the healing time is also much longer. As Jane says, "Lips are a process, not a procedure."

Your lips will feel sore and very dry for a while after each treatment, so this is one area where Jane says you can go ahead and splurge on the ointment. Apply it several times a day with a cotton swab for at least two weeks and don't let your lips get dry. She advises that you dab the ointment on, rather than rubbing it in.

For the first few days, Jane recommends that you brush your teeth with water only and not use any whitening products. As with all of these procedures, stay out of the sun and swimming pools and don't wear any lip products for the minimum two-week period. After that, avoid lip products that contain glycolic (fruit) and alpha- or beta-hydroxy acids.

For a full month after each treatment, you need to avoid anything that can irritate your lips. This includes eating greasy or salty foods and allowing any kind of friction; that means no wiping your mouth and *no kissing* or other oral acts of intimacy (wink, wink!). Then, once you're all healed up from the first treatment, you have to go through that all over again.

The most common side effects of lip tattoos are fever blisters and hyperpigmentation, which is a darkening of the skin due to an increase of melanin. If that happens, it can often be corrected with another color treatment, but not always. If you already have hyperpigmentation on your lips from trauma or sun damage, or naturally darker lips due to your ethnicity, you may not be a good candidate for lip tattooing.

AREOLAS

Areola restoration can also take up to three separate treatments to create the full effect. The coloring will be inconsistent if there's a lot of scar tissue—either too dark or too light—during various stages of the healing process. You have to trust that your artist used the right shades and that it will all come out fine in the end.

Ointment should be used sparingly; just enough to keep the area protected. When you shower, avoid using very hot water or allowing the water to flow directly onto the tattoo. Whenever you can, going braless or even topless will allow the tattoo to breathe and encourage healing.

Scabbing is to be expected, and it's important that you don't pick at the scabs or remove any skin or pigment flakes. They'll fall off on their own when they're ready; forcing them to come off too soon can pull color. Even so, some color loss is normal and can be corrected during the follow-up visits.

ᎧᏣ Lifetime Maintenance

While there will probably come a time when you'll need your tattoos touched up to restore their original color depth, keeping them protected from the sun and harsh chemicals will help lengthen the time between touch-ups.

Other than that, your cosmetic tattoos become a part of you and can make you feel more beautiful and confident for many years to come.

Granted, not everyone reading this book can get tattooed by Jane Adler, but if you seek out an artist with the same dedication and care as Jane, you're sure to be happy with your results.

the beauty of scarification

It's easy to initially recoil at the thought of scarification when you think about the process it takes to get there. For some reason, it seems much more dramatic than driving a steel bar through your flesh or puncturing the surface millions of times. It doesn't help if you've seen documentaries of tribal rituals that involve repeatedly slicing the skin of children with a dirty razor blade as a rite of passage into adulthood. But modern scarification really isn't that much different from other forms of permanent body art, and the results can be just as beautiful.

The most intriguing part about this particular art form, though, is its unpredictable nature. That's what some people find most appealing about it—kind of like playing poker, only you don't usually find out what kind of hand you had until the game is over, so you're playing blind. Are you feeling lucky?

✎ Do Not Try This at Home

I think it goes without saying, though, that scarification is a very dangerous procedure—especially in the wrong hands—and a lot of things can go wrong. It's imperative that you find an artist who is both qualified and experienced. That's not an easy thing to do, since there aren't a lot of people offering scarification services, and those who do don't get a lot of practice if there isn't much demand for it in their area. Most of them are primarily tattoo or piercing artists and offer scarification on the side.

While there are many different methods by which to injure the skin and produce a scar, not all of them are safe or offer the artist a measure of control over the design. The two safest and most common methods are cutting and branding, which will be covered here. Both methods have their share of pros and cons, so this is the best place to compare the two before you decide which way to go.

Since I've not had the benefit of actually experiencing a scarification procedure myself, I spoke to Jesse Villemaire at Thrive Studios in Cambridge, Ontario, Canada, to get the scoop on the inner workings of this unique body modification. Jesse has been a scarification artist since 2003 and is already making a name for himself as one of the best in the biz.

✎ Cutting

Jesse does all of his scarification work via the cutting method because he feels that it gives him much more control to create intricate patterns. I want to say, right from the start, that this is completely different from the kind of cutting that self-harmers do. People who cut themselves for an emotional release aren't worried about making pretty patterns, and people who want pretty patterns aren't in it for the pain. Jesse does see many former cutters, though, who are ready to put that life behind them by getting a scar that they can associate good memories with.

"I'm into it for the art and not for satisfying the needs of a self-cutter. Most self-harmers will not seek out a professional to do scarification on them. This is one of the reasons I like to meet with a client beforehand to assess what they are hoping to get out of this experience."

—JESSE V.

✎ Understanding the Risks

Before he begins working on a client, Jesse likes to sit down and talk with them about what they're looking for. During that time, he'll explain the process and make sure that this is what they really want. An important part of this conversation is also discussing the risks and making sure the client understands the serious nature of what they are about to undergo.

The biggest risk is infection, and with this kind of procedure, a small infection can turn very bad, very quickly. Large flesh openings are an open invitation to staph bacteria and other harmful germs. Damaged tissue can become gangrenous, and some infections can spread to the bloodstream and affect the whole body. But having an artist like Jesse, who is impeccably clean, lowers that risk to almost nothing. One of his clients, Shawn Johnston, learned how to clean and sterilize equipment at another shop where he used to work, and even he says, "What Jesse does is so far above and beyond what most other shops do when it comes to tidiness and sterilization."

But once you walk out the door, keeping your cutting clean is your responsibility, so a really hygienic artist can't be blamed if the client doesn't take care of their work. As long as you and your artist both take the necessary steps to be as clean as humanly possible, everything usually heals up just fine. Jesse has many satisfied clients with beautiful scars that testify to his immaculate skills.

Another risk you take when it comes to this artistic venue is not knowing the end results. Some people scar really well, while others— damn their overly healthy immune systems—will simply heal over and have very little to show for the time and pain that went into the design. During the consultation, Jesse will also look at any existing scars on the client to see how their body naturally reacts to injury and how well they scar. Sometimes it's decided that they would actually be better suited for a tattoo because of the size or design they're looking for. But if the client is ready to proceed, it's on to the drawing board.

> "Scarification is one of the only body modifications in which your own body has complete control over the end results. It's a real gamble; I can cut the same design on multiple people in the exact same spot on their body, and it can heal completely different on every one of them."
>
> —JESSE V.

ℰ From Paper to Flesh

Once the design is approved on paper, a stencil is made to transfer onto the client's skin. This is the same kind of stencil that is used before a tattoo, so the client can view the outlines ahead of time and approve size, placement, and angle. There's no going back once the skin is cut, so it's important that everything is just right.

The tools Jesse uses are very basic—a scalpel handle and several sterile blades. Everything else he uses is all about protecting himself and his client: disposable gloves, disposable sleeves, a disposable apron, a face mask, antiseptic skin prep, and sterile gauze. The blades aren't all the same; they come in different sizes and shapes. Jesse chooses his blades according to the particular design he's doing—to create the best effect— just as a painter would use more than one brush to complete a painting.

Once Jesse starts cutting, it's extremely gentle at first. He does a very shallow carving along the outer lines of the design; just enough to break the skin. The pain of this initial cut is similar to getting tattooed— not excruciating but definitely noticeable. This step helps to create a more stable stencil line that can't be wiped away, and it opens the skin just

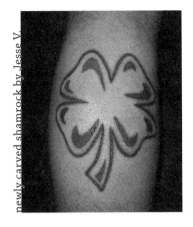
newly carved shamrock by Jesse V.

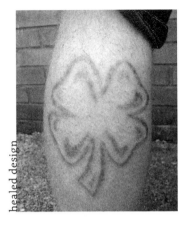
healed design

enough to get the full benefit of the topical anesthetic Jesse then applies. The anesthetic spray serves two purposes: One, obviously, is to lessen pain for the client, but it also contains epinephrine, which shrinks the blood vessels and minimizes bleeding, making a cleaner canvas for Jesse to work on.

> "On a pain scale of one to ten, I'd give getting cut a five. The numbing spray Jesse uses really helps. Plus, whenever I go in for scar work, there's usually someone there getting tattooed, so I just listen to the sound of the buzzing and it feels pretty much the same as getting tattooed."
>
> **—SHAWN JOHNSTON,**
> **HAPPY CLIENT OF JESSE VILLEMAIRE**

Jesse is very meticulous in his art, and working clean is important to working safe so that he can see how deeply he's cutting. This is the part that requires great skill, because the depth to which the blade cuts into your skin can greatly affect the results, good or bad. Too shallow, and the skin won't separate enough to produce sufficient scarring. Too deep, and you could end up in the hospital.

The process of cutting the skin is actually done in small steps, carefully slicing short sections multiple times to achieve the right depth and width across the entire design. Some liken the feeling to getting a series of paper cuts. Surgical blades are designed to make maximum penetration with minimal tissue damage. People who attempt this kind of procedure using household razors can really hurt someone, because there are many microscopic serrations on a blade that may look smooth to the naked eye, but those serrations rip and tear through tissue like a hacksaw.

∽ Don't Hold Your Breath

Cutting a design from beginning to end takes just a little bit longer than a comparably sized tattoo. Sitting for hours having your skin sliced open can be a little rough on the nervous system. Plus, the endorphin rush from this process tends to be stronger than the one that results from getting a tattoo, which for some is half the thrill of the experience. But it wouldn't take much for a client to pass out from the resultant high, especially if they hadn't eaten properly before the appointment. It's important to have a small, healthy meal about an hour before the cutting begins to regulate your blood sugar.

Breathing is also important. During moments of intense pain, it's a natural reaction to want to hold your breath, which really only makes it worse. There's a reason pregnant women learn the art of breathing to ease pain during labor. Unfortunately, there aren't any Lamaze classes for scarification, but the concept is still relevant: Inhale slowly through the nose and exhale slowly through the mouth. Deep, slow breaths will relax your muscles and raise your pain threshold. Not that getting a scar is an excruciating experience, but we all reach a point when the pain becomes more intense, and you have to be able to push through it if the design isn't finished yet.

> *"Breathing is very important. I've met many clients in the past that will continue to hold their breath when they get a piercing, tattoo, or scar done. Usually this results in the*

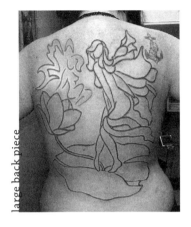

large back piece

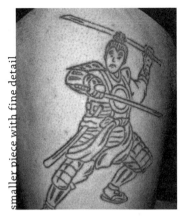

smaller piece with fine detail

client passing out. I just like to ask a lot of questions that the client has to answer to keep their mind active and off of the procedure itself. Once we're talking and joking around, it usually helps ease their mind."

—JESSE V.

If you've chosen a design that is very large or very detailed, it's possible to split the process up into more than one session. This way you're not putting so much stress on your body all at once, and you have some time to heal in between sessions. Always make arrangements to split up your sessions ahead of time.

∽ Skinned Alive

The most dangerous part of any cutting process is the removal of surface skin. Our skin is actually an organ that is designed to work as a whole; when part of that network is missing, the entire system suffers until it's able to repair itself. It's also the only barrier between us and the rest of the world, and our main defense against the invasion of antigens. So this has to be taken very seriously and done with great care.

Jesse tries to avoid the need for skin removal as much as possible by forming a sufficiently wide line through cutting only. But from time to time, a particular design may necessitate the need to amputate a small area of skin. Jesse knows the ramifications of this and fully prepares his clients by warning them of the increased risk of infection or injury. Because he's so safety conscious and his clients are so well informed, even these areas usually heal up without incident.

๑ The Importance of Aftercare

Aftercare is a bit of a balancing act—you want it to heal, but you also want it to scar. This is why some scarification artists will recommend prolonging the healing process by irritating the wound with lemon juice or hydrogen peroxide, or scrubbing it with a new toothbrush. These methods aren't necessarily bad or dangerous, but they may not be necessary. Most of Jesse's clients find that their designs scar up just fine without any further injury to the wound, so he doesn't recommend any of these methods.

What he does recommend is the "leave it alone" method, meaning that as long as you keep yourself healthy and keep the wound clean, your body will generally take care of the rest. This also helps to achieve a more uniform scar and protects you from serious injury and infection.

Every artist is going to have their own personal recommendations on how to care for your wounds. If you trusted them enough to cut you in the first place, you can probably trust them to know how to treat their work. If you encounter any problems, call them—don't wait for something to progress to a dangerous situation because you don't want to "bother" your artist or because you think you don't have time. If you're having second thoughts about the qualifications of your "artist," then at least find someone that can help you, or go to the doctor, especially if you think you might be developing an infection.

๑ How Branding Compares to Cutting

The end result of branding is very similar to that of cutting; the major difference is the process used to get there. As I mentioned earlier, there

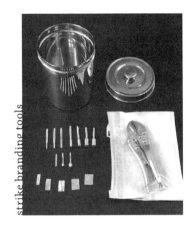
strike branding tools

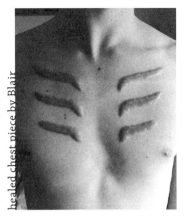
healed chest piece by Blair

are pros and cons to both methods, and it's up to you to decide which one sounds more appealing.

The process of branding involves cauterizing the skin with intense heat. That may sound really painful, especially if you've ever burned your hand on a hot stove or gotten a similar surface burn. But the goal with branding isn't a surface burn, which wouldn't produce any scarring anyway. Branding devices attain temperatures in excess of one thousand degrees Fahrenheit, and when they are placed firmly against the skin, they quickly produce third-degree burns.

While that actually sounds worse than a surface burn, the advantage is that it also destroys the nerve endings that transmit pain. Most victims of accidental third-degree burns describe the feeling as numbness. When my husband was a teenager, he burned most of his leg in an accidental fire. He had no skin left over much of his leg, and he doesn't recall ever being in considerable pain. He described the experience as uncomfortable at most. So, even though third-degree burns sound horribly painful, it's actually more painful to receive a superficial burn.

That's not to say that third-degree burns aren't physically traumatic, though, because they certainly are. That kind of intense tissue destruction over large areas can send a person into shock. Granted, most aesthetic brandings aren't that large, and the artist *should* be aware of what is and isn't a reasonable amount to be done in one sitting, but everyone has a different tolerance level.

One risk with some branding methods is that even once the heated device has been removed from the skin, the tissue can continue to burn for up to twenty-four hours after the procedure. Second-degree burns, which are very painful, can develop around the initial brand. The scars that develop as a result of branding are generally more significant than those from cutting and will form about three or four times the width of the initial line.

The same risks of infection exist with branding as with cutting. It's extremely important that the area be kept clean, since dead tissue is a feast for bacteria.

Human aesthetic branding isn't done with an iron prod that's been sitting in hot coals, like what farmers use to mark their livestock. Yes, I've seen videos of frat boys and other idiots branding their butts that way for the entertainment of onlookers, but that's not how the professionals do it. Professional branding is a gentler but much slower application, and it can be done a few different ways.

Strike branding is the closest to animal branding in that a piece of heated metal is placed firmly against the skin until the desired burn is attained, which usually takes only a couple of seconds. A thin, flat length of sheet metal is usually heated with a propane torch, and short lines are made, one at a time, until the entire design has been burned. It's a slow process, and you're usually limited to large, geometric shapes and simple patterns.

Electrocautery branding is a method that requires a special tool—also called an electrocautery—that uses an electrical current to heat a small wire at the tip. The current heats the wire and the wire is then placed on the skin. The current is intermittent, so the tip doesn't stay hot constantly and the brand has to be done one tiny section at a time. It's an excruciatingly slow process, but it does provide a means of creating slightly more intricate designs, since it's easier to make rounded shapes than to make just straight lines.

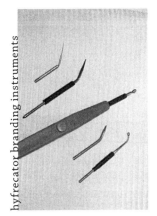
hyfrecator branding instruments

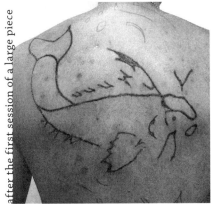
after the first session of a large piece

Hyfrecator branding is also referred to as electrosurgery. It's similar to the electrocautery but more advanced and much faster. Instead of using electricity to heat the tip and then deliver heat to the skin, electricity is delivered directly to the skin by the tip of the probe. It is highly directional and burns only the tissue it's directed at, leaving the surrounding tissue safe from additional burns. This also minimizes the extended formation of scarring beyond the width of the initial burn line, so tighter and more intricate designs are possible.

> *TIP: One drawback to branding versus cutting is the acrid smell of burning skin, which a lot of people can't stomach. The fumes that are produced by the vaporized flesh also contain biological matter that can potentially include harmful bacteria, so artists usually wear a ventilated safety mask to protect themselves against those vapors. The client is also offered a filtration mask to help reduce exposure to the smell. Proper ventilation and air filtration are also important to keeping the air as clean and fresh as possible, but some odor is bound to permeate the room at some point.*

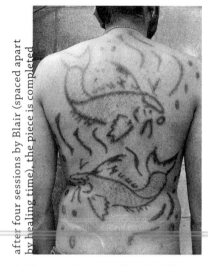

after four sessions by Blair (spaced apart by healing time), the piece is completed

Unfortunately, medical devices such as the electrocautery and hyfrecator are not approved for use by nonmedical personnel in some areas, depending on state or local regulation laws. This is why you don't see many branding artists offering these services in the United States. One of the most highly respected branding artists who uses the hyfrecator on his clients is Blair. His shop, Burned Alive, is located in Toronto, Ontario, Canada. If you want a brand done by this method, it just might be worth a trip across the border.

Canada offers scarification artists more opportunities to experiment and evolve the art because the industry isn't regulated, which isn't necessarily a good thing. Reputable artists like Jesse and Blair impose strict sanitation rules on themselves without needing regulation, but others can take advantage of that freedom and cause a lot of harm. It's very important that you make sure that your chosen artist is highly concerned about personal cleanliness and client safety, whether the laws tells them to be so or not.

Because there are so few reputable scarification artists out there, the ones doing the best work are a tight community and communicate among themselves to continue improving their techniques. You're best off choosing an artist within that community, and you will probably need to be willing to travel. Some of Jesse's friends and personal favorites are Ron Garza, Brian Decker, Wayde Dunn, John Joyce, Ryan Ouellette, and, of course, Blair. Even if you can't personally get work done by one of these artists, I would trust any one of them to steer you in the right direction toward finding someone equally qualified.

implants and extreme modifications

Due to the fact that implants are considered surgical procedures and that most laws in the United States don't allow nonmedical personnel to perform them, this chapter will just give you a basic overview of these kinds of procedures. If you want to get an implant, you'll have to research laws in your area, and you may even have to travel abroad to find a qualified artist. Such qualified artists are few and far between, so it's very important that you do extensive research before getting any of the following procedures.

∾ Transdermal Implants

I already covered microdermal implants in the piercing section because they really do qualify more as a piercing than as an actual implant, but there is a very similar procedure called a transdermal implant. But because of the complexity involved in comparison with a microdermal, transdermals belong in this section.

The main similarity between transdermals and microdermals is that they both have one part that exists under the skin and then a short, threaded screw assembly that protrudes outward, which can then be used to attach a variety of gems, spikes, or even horns.

True transdermal implants are quite dangerous and involve a lot more tissue than microdermals, but they do tend to be more stable once healed. That stability also means that if you ever want to remove the implant, you'll have to have another surgical procedure to cut it out.

Instead of making a single hole, transdermals require making two holes, at least an inch apart, which are then used to insert the jewelry base, which is typically a long, flat bar. Then all the connective tissue between the two points has to be loosened up to allow for the base insertion, so a dermal separator is used to pry the layers of skin apart. Then the base is inserted into one hole and threaded through to the second, and the protruding screw is pushed up through the second hole. The first hole is then usually sewn back together with stitches so that it can heal.

⁊ Subdermal Implants

Subdermals don't have anything that protrudes out from the skin, as they are completely encased underneath the dermis. It's the implant itself that lifts the skin up from underneath and leaves a three-dimensional marking that creates the visual effect.

An incision is made in the skin with a scalpel, and then the connective tissue is loosened with a dermal separator in order to create a pocket in which the implant can be placed. Then the incision is stitched back together, and that's really the only part that needs to heal.

Implants can come in a variety of shapes, depending on the effect you want. The three-dimensional shape is placed under the skin for aesthetic purposes, either alone or in conjunction with other body art such as a tattoo. I met Jamie Holtfreter—a piercer at Artkore Tattoo in Normal, Illinois—at the Hell City tattoo convention, and she had a cupcake shape implanted in one hand and an ice cream cone in the other, which both went very well with the Strawberry Shortcake tattoos she had all down her arm.

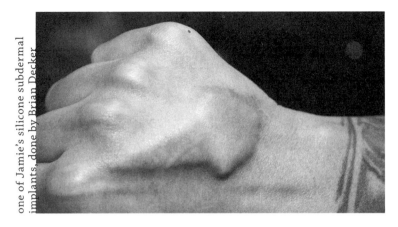

one of Jamie's silicone subdermal implants, done by Brian Decker

Jamie's implants were done by Brian Decker, a highly respected piercer and modification artist who owns Pure Body Arts in Brooklyn, New York. She said that the incision made for inserting the implant is actually quite small—about half an inch in width. The silicone implants are squishy, so they're squeezed into a smaller size before being inserted through the incision. Once underneath the skin, they puff back up and take their full form.

On a scale of one to ten, Jamie said the pain level of getting the implants done was definitely a high nine. She was sore and bruised for a couple of weeks afterward as well. But she has had them for two years now and has had very little shifting and no complications with them. Having them done by someone as skilled as Brian Decker definitely helps with the success rate.

> "If you want implants, I say go for it, but do your research. Nowadays people think that they can do them just because they know the process in theory, but that doesn't make them an expert. I'm an experienced body piercer and you don't see me offering implants. It's a specialized skill."
>
> **—JAMIE HOLTFRETER**

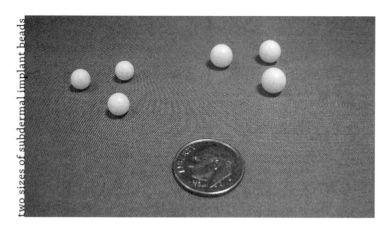

Other times, implants are used for physical reasons, as with genital beading or genital ribs, in which small round beads or barbells are placed along the shaft of the penis to create a permanent bumpy texture.

Implants have to be biocompatible, so molded silicone, PTFE, and titanium are the most popular materials used to make objects for implanting.

Even though the process of getting the implant is relatively simple, each one comes with a relatively long list of associated risks, which increase over time; the longer the implant resides under your skin, the more likely you are to develop some kind of complication, some of which can be very dangerous. This is why going to an experienced artist is so important: You need to be fully aware of all the potential problems you may face not just now, but many months or years down the road.

ঙ Extreme Modifications

There are many more interesting but dangerous procedures that people can do to their bodies in the name of self-expression. Tongue splitting, ear pointing, and tooth filing are just a few of the modifications that are gaining popularity as more people attempt to push the envelope of body modification to greater heights.

For some, the appeal of body art is that it enables them to be separated from the normal crowd; the more accepted and mainstream a procedure becomes, the less attractive it is to those who seek to stand out. These are the people who have been opening doors of opportunity for expression by inventing new and exciting ways to enhance the body. But they're also the same people who are experimenting with some very dangerous ideas that could do irreparable harm to those who are impulsive and inexperienced.

There's a reason why you'll usually see the same names in the news when a new, outlandish kind of body modification is attempted. Modifiers themselves who have been experts in their field for many years are usually the ones who will guinea pig themselves out to experiment with something new.

Even Shannon Larratt, founder of and former writer for the extreme body modification website BMEzine.com, while taking part in the world's first eyeball-tattooing experiment, had this to say to the general public:

"I really have to emphasize again that the procedure was extensively researched and done by people who were aware of the risks and possible complications and that it should not be casually attempted. Now that this experiment has been started, please wait for us to either heal or go blind before trying it!"

So leave the extreme stuff to the experts and be content with the many beautiful and *safe* ways there are to express yourself.

mehndi: the art of henna painting

Mehndi is a beautiful, temporary body art that is created by using a powerful dye that's derived from the *Lawsonia inermis* (henna) bush. The leaves are dried and crushed into a powder, which is then mixed with other ingredients to form a paste. The paste is applied to the skin and allowed to set; upon removal, a stain is left behind that will remain for approximately two weeks. It's safe, temporary but long-lasting, and a lot of fun.

The use of henna has been around for at least five thousand years, but not always for decorative purposes. The exact point of origin has been debated, but we do know that evidence of henna use goes back to ancient Egypt, where it was used for pharmaceutical purposes and to stain the fingers and toes of the pharaohs prior to mummification. At some point, it was introduced in India, where it evolved into more elaborate designs and became an integral part of their culture and rituals. From there, it slowly made its way to the West, where it has been adapted purely for aesthetics and artistic enjoyment.

Although henna art is sometimes referred to as a "tattoo," it is really nothing of the sort. It doesn't require puncturing the skin and it isn't permanent. It is simply a thick dye that stains the surface of the skin and penetrates deeply enough to remain for a while, until the epidermis has regenerated enough times to exfoliate the cells that were colored. The more you wash and scrub your skin, the quicker this will happen.

∽ Color Warning!

Naked henna (meaning natural in its purest form) does not come in a variety of colors. Henna powder is green—the paste can be anywhere between a dark green and a dark brown—and the stain it leaves behind is a burnt-rust color that usually turns a shade of dark orange or brown. The actual shade of the stain depends on your skin tone and the strength of the paste itself.

Colored henna is not natural, so there's no guarantee that you won't have a reaction to the synthetic materials used to create the colors. Companies that sell the dyes may claim that they are derived from "organic compounds," but that doesn't mean they're safe. Take PPD (short for paraphenylenediamine), for example, which is an aromatic amine. Aromatic amines are defined as "organic chemicals that are used in the manufacture of industrial chemicals, pesticides, and dyes and are also naturally occurring."

PPD is typically used in fabric and fur dye, printer inks, and black rubber. NIOSH (the National Institute for Occupational Safety and Health) lists PPD as a hazardous chemical. Permanent hair dyes often use PPD, but the packaging has to include printed warnings about the risk of severe allergic reactions.

If you've ever colored your own hair, you've seen the "magic" of PPD. You usually have to squeeze a tube of color into a bottle of developer. At first, it barely has any color at all, but after a few minutes it can turn dark brown, bright red, or even pitch-black. Ever wonder why it does that? It's because of the PPD. It's colorless until it comes into contact with the air, which causes a chemical reaction called oxidation. Oxidation is the same thing that causes your apple slices to turn brown and turned the Statue of Liberty green. That oxidation process is what gives PPD its coveted, rich, coal-black coloring.

> *"Hair color can cause an allergic reaction which, in certain rare cases, can be severe. This product contains ingredients which may cause skin irritation on certain individuals and a preliminary test according to accompanying directions should first be made."*
> **—WARNING LABEL ON GARNIER HAIR COLOR, WHICH CONTAINS PPD**

Now that we've established that PPD is a dangerous, caustic substance, it doesn't sound like something you'd want to put on your skin, does it? And yet some companies and individuals are adding PPD—in *high* concentrations, no less—to henna paste and marketing it as "black henna," to be used for skin design. Why? Because people want their henna tattoos to look more like real ones, and the black color gives that illusion. Plus, black henna sets faster, making it easier for the so-called "artist" to make a quick buck.

Black henna tattoos are the cause of dozens of serious chemical burns every year, which happen mostly to children who get the designs while on vacation. The main offenders in this scheme are the ones working at carnivals, beaches, and other temporary establishments. By the time the PPD starts to burn your skin, the transient vendor who applied it has moved on to another location.

In April 2008, eleven- and fifteen-year-old sisters Emily and Megan Riley were both permanently scarred by the henna "tattoos" they received while vacationing in Branson, Missouri. In June of the same year, ten-year-old Charlie Wallace's arm was burned by the black henna he got on his arm while on holiday in Marmaris, Turkey. That same month, Jayden

Robertson, only six years old, began to blister from the henna that had been applied to his skin while vacationing in Kuta, Bali.

Not all reactions to black henna are immediate. In July 2008, seven-year-old Taylor Leslie-Aune received a henna tattoo at the four-star hotel where his family was staying in Mexico. The tattoo was normal throughout the vacation and faded over the following weeks, as expected. But once the original design was gone, it reappeared in the form of an angry welt in the exact shape of the tattoo. In October, Vinnie England—just three years old—was left with a permanent scar in the shape of Bart Simpson from the henna he received while vacationing in Benidorm, Spain. These stories are just a few that actually made it to the news; this kind of thing happens all too often and it needs to stop. When someone doesn't even care that they're hurting children, it reaches an entirely new level of disgrace.

If you go to a vendor and you aren't sure what kind of henna they're using, ask if you can take a close look at it; it should be a dark green or greenish-brown in color. Take a sniff; true henna paste doesn't smell good, but it doesn't smell like chemicals either. It usually has a mixture of scents, like eucalyptus, grass, and dirt, with a touch of a pungent moldlike or tobaccolike smell. Again, not a pleasant aroma to most people, but earthy nevertheless. It definitely shouldn't be black, and it shouldn't smell harsh or sharp like a chemical. If the vendor tells you it will turn black, even if they insist it's safe, walk away.

Henna, in its truly natural state, mixed only with skin-safe ingredients, is beautiful just as it is. The earth-tone colors it produces when it stains the skin should be appreciated without trying to change them. Not everything needs to be westernized or modernized; enjoy taking part in something with a rich history and beautiful cultural and ritualistic significance.

ꙮ Let's Paint!

Now that we got all the serious stuff out of the way, let's move on to the fun part! Making and applying henna is simple and a lot of fun. And unlike many other types of body art, this one you *can* do at home!

The first thing you need to decide is whether you want to buy premade paste or make your own. Making your own is a bit of a complicated process, but it's also a fun one if you see it as just another part of the craft. If you're the type that gets more joy from making your own cake than from buying one already made, then you might also enjoy making your own henna paste. If not, there's no shame in buying a premade paste. Just make sure it doesn't contain any harmful ingredients. My favorite premixed henna paste is made by an online company called Natural Expressions. I've been ordering from them for years and have always been happy with their products, even though I'm not fond of the fact that they also sell tattoo and piercing kits. Do me a favor and ignore those pages, okay?

Anyway, if you decide to make your own paste, there are some things you'll want to know first before you proceed.

✑ Making Henna Paste

The first thing you need to know is that not all henna is created equal. You already know that henna is made from the crushed, dried leaves of the *Lawsonia inermis* bush. But what you probably don't know is that the henna bush grows in many different regions of India, Pakistan, and northern Africa. Different regions have different climates, some wet, some dry. The type of climate that henna is grown in greatly affects the levels of lawsone—also known as hennotannic acid—in the leaves. The level of tannins in the leaves determines the level of stain they will produce on the skin.

Years ago, when I was first learning how to make henna paste, I ran out of powder and tried to find a local source rather than ordering it online and waiting for it to be delivered. I found some at a nearby health food store; it was in a large container and sold by weight, so there was nothing to indicate that it was meant for any specific purpose. But I figured *henna's henna, right?* Wrong. I still don't know what kind of henna that was, but it wasn't meant for mehndi. After I spent hours creating a paste with the powder and using up my other ingredients, it left behind absolutely no stain at all. Lesson learned—only buy henna that is specifically marketed for mehndi.

In addition to finding the right kind of henna, it's also important that it's fresh. If you buy it from the shelf of an Indian grocery store and it looks like it's covered in dust and hasn't been touched in a year, it's probably stale. Stale henna doesn't stain well at all. The best way to know whether your henna powder is fresh or not is by sight and smell. It should be rich green in color and smell like freshly mown grass. If it looks dull or brown and smells like rotting hay, it's gone bad.

Now you have another decision to make: Do you want to use presifted henna or sift it yourself? Sifting henna is a messy process and I highly recommend buying it presifted. And yes, it is important that the powder is sifted, because it can contain a lot of twigs and other impurities that will adversely affect the outcome of the paste.

If you really want to have the full mehndi experience and sift your own powder, work at a table and cover it with newspaper; things are about to get very messy. You will need a tall, sturdy plastic cup, a rubber band, and an old pair of panty hose. Put some of the powder inside the cup, stretch a square of panty hose over the end and secure it with the rubber band as tightly as you can get it. Then turn the cup upside down and start shaking, collecting the sifted powder in a plastic bowl. A very fine cloud of henna will slowly build around you; the longer you sift, the bigger the cloud. I think I was cleaning bits of green powder out of tiny nooks and crannies of my kitchen for a week the last time I sifted my own powder— that's why it was the last time.

TIP: You always want to use plastic or glass bowls, containers, and utensils when working with henna. The acidic properties of henna paste can tarnish metal, so you want to use something that's inert.

Once you have a fine, sifted powder to work with, it's time to start mixing up the paste. It's not an exact science—there are a lot of different things you can use to make henna paste, but each thing serves a different purpose.

- **ACID:** Your paste will need some kind of acidic element to draw out the lawsone from the crushed leaves and encourage the tannins to absorb into the skin. What kind of acid you use is your choice—lemon juice, lime juice, and vinegar are the top three options. Incidentally, lime juice is the most acidic of the three.

- **TERPENES:** Particularly monoterpene alcohol, a substance found in some essential oils, serves as a catalyst to encourage a deeper, darker stain. Tea tree oil and lavender essential oil are two of the most effective substances that contain terpenes.

- **SUGAR:** This makes the paste stick to the skin better and crack less as it dries. Honey, glycerin, corn syrup, and even granulated sugar are the most popular options.

- **FRAGRANCE:** If the essential oil you added for terpenes isn't enough to mask the smell of the henna (which some people find appealing, while others do not), then you may want to add an additional ingredient for fragrance. A few drops of some other kind of essential oil or extract you like should do the trick.

> *TIP: If you're going to use your henna paste on a child (never put henna on an infant) then you should omit the essential oils. A child's skin is very sensitive and essential oils can be harsh, even in small amounts. It would also be good to use a very mild acidic ingredient.*

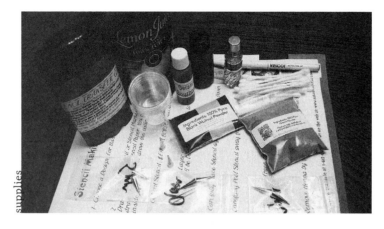

How much of each thing you add to your recipe is pretty much up to you. Your acidic ingredient is the main element, so you want to add that first; keep adding until you've reached a consistency similar to that of peanut butter. Then you add just enough sugar to smooth it out and make it more like cake frosting. Since your essential oils will consist of only a few drops, they won't do much to change the viscosity. Other than following those basic rules, you can just sort of "wing it," but always write down what you've tried so if you create the perfect recipe, you'll be able to duplicate it later.

> *TIP: It's a good idea to heat the lemon juice before adding it to the henna powder, to assist the process of releasing the tannins. Some henna artists will also put the finished paste under a mild heat source, like a desk lamp, for a few hours afterward.*

There are many different ingredients you can play and experiment with to see what works best for you. Other things you can try if you're feeling froggy are: wine, coffee, tea, tamarind, ground cloves, citric acid, and whatever else you feel like throwing in for good measure! If the paste becomes too thin, add some more henna powder. If it's too thick, thin it out with more liquid. As long as you start with the right ingredients, you really can't go wrong!

Once your paste is mixed, it needs to set for a minimum of two hours and as long as a full day. Place plastic wrap over it and leave it alone. The longer it sets, the more tannins can be extracted from the leaves. It should reach its full potential by the time it's twenty-four hours old.

↜ Dispensing Options

Once your paste is ready to go, you need to have something to dispense and apply it with. There are several options for doing this, and there's no right or wrong way—just personal preference.

Little plastic bottles with metal tips are probably the easiest method and best for the inexperienced henna artist. The applicator bottles come with a capacity to hold as little as half an ounce of paste and as much as two ounces. Anything larger than a two-ounce bottle would be difficult to hold and control. Tips come in a variety of sizes, too, with ultrafine tips having a five-millimeter opening and increasing gradually to as large as nine millimeters. Different designs and patterns require different line widths, so it's good to have several sizes on hand. Then all you have to do is put the paste in the bottle, turn it upside down, and squeeze to apply the henna.

Syringes can also be used for superfine lines, but they can be used only with very thin and stringy henna, which requires a more advanced user to be able to control it. Syringe tips are sometimes available with attachments for plastic applicator bottles.

Piping bags are one of my favorites, but they also take a little practice. They're the same kind of thing that cake decorators use to apply icing, but you want to use smaller—and probably disposable—versions. Some disposable piping bags are made of heavy plastic and are stiff, but you want to find ones that are soft and easy to manipulate. Ten-inch bags are plenty large for applying henna, since working with smaller amounts will give you greater control. You can cut a tiny hole at the end of the piping bag or you can use a variety of decorator tips, which are held in place with couplers. Small pointed cellophane bags used for gifting food items work well, too!

Another option that is very similar to the piping bag method is the cone. A cone is shaped just like a piping bag—pointed at one end and large at the other. You can make your own cones easily and inexpensively. Cellophane gift wrap, plastic freezer bags, and even Mylar all work well to create cones. Just cut out a triangle of your selected material, roll it up in a cone shape with a nice, tight tip at the bottom, and tape it together. Voilà! Instant henna cone, ready for use.

If you want to try something different, you can even use brushes to apply the paste. Oil-painting brushes come in a wide variety of shapes and sizes and work very well for applying henna for larger designs. Since it's all temporary, it never hurts to try something just for the fun of it. Don't be afraid to be creative.

✺ Preparing Your Design

Once you've got your henna in a dispenser of some sort, you are ready to begin applying the henna. The skin area you will be applying it to should be cleaned with an alcohol prep pad to remove any oils and dirt that can hinder the staining process. If the person is hairy or fuzzy in the area where you'll be painting, you may want to use a new, disposable razor to gently remove the hair. The paste needs to have direct contact with the skin in order to stain it, and even tiny hairs can lift the paste above the skin's surface.

What kind of design or pattern you do is up to you or the person you're applying it to. There are the traditional paisley designs like the ones Indian women apply to their hands and feet for wedding ceremonies. You can find free patterns online or buy books that include mehndi patterns. You can also use regular tattoo patterns and drawings. Or you can just use your imagination and freehand something unique, using a combination of lines, swirls, dots, and other simple shapes. As long as the design is within your personal skill level, you can do almost anything you want. Henna is a great way for people to try out a tattoo idea they're considering, before making it permanent.

If you decide to use a pattern, you'll need to transfer the pattern to the skin unless you're adept at drawing and can follow a simple pattern fairly well. If you need to transfer the pattern, use Spirit Master hectograph paper (the thermal kind won't work unless you have a Thermofax) to trace your design and then apply it to the skin. Putting a very thin application of something moist and sticky on the skin, like gel deodorant or personal lubricating gel, will help the transfer take better. Be sure that neither of these products is used directly on another person unless it is new and you plan to dispose of it afterward. Otherwise, first put some on a paper towel and then use that to apply the gel to the skin. Then press your carbon paper up against the skin (carbon side down, of course!) and you'll get a purple copy of your design that you can trace over with the henna.

> *TIP: Where you decide to draw a henna design is optional, but there's a reason why the hands and feet are such popular locations. Skin that is rough and dry is also more absorbent and can pull a darker stain than other areas, like arms or legs. If you're applying it to a less absorbent location, just take all the other measures you can for a good stain, and you should still be happy with the results.*

✑ Ready, Set, Draw!

You've got your design plan down, and now you're ready to start applying the henna to the skin. I always do a couple of practice lines on a paper towel first, just to make sure it's at the consistency I want to work with and it's dispensing smoothly. Then, when I know I'm ready, I move on to the client.

Squeeze slowly and steadily and work in small sections if you need to. Breaks in lines won't hurt the overall stain as long as you start a new

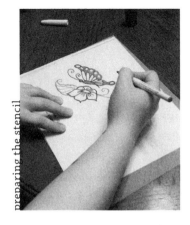
preparing the stencil

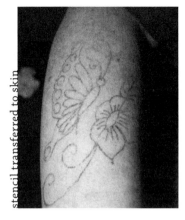
stencil transferred to skin

line where the last one ended. Short cracks in the henna can be filled in. It doesn't all have to look like one smooth line. That comes with practice, but the henna will stain the skin it's touching, one way or another.

Be aware that a good, strong henna will begin to stain the skin immediately, so if you mess up, you need to be prepared to clean it as quickly as possible. Having some cotton swabs already premoistened with rubbing alcohol can help to quickly clean up a mistake.

✎ Dry and Set

Once you have finished drawing on your design, the paste needs to set so that the lawsone can bond with the keratin in the skin, which is what helps create a deep, lasting stain.

Making sure the paste is dry is the first step. Using a hair dryer or having a heat lamp placed over the area can help accomplish this more quickly and effectively, but you want to be careful to not let it dry too much. Henna tends to crack and pull apart when it's very dry, and those "holes" in the pattern can leave a blank spot where there should be a stain. So let the paste dry just enough to be firm to the touch, but not brittle. If you accidentally let it dry too much, fill in any cracks with fresh paste and begin the drying process again.

When the paste is at the firm-but-not-brittle stage, you will need to seal it. Henna needs to stay on the skin for several hours to achieve the best

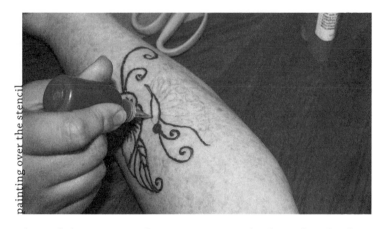

painting over the stencil

results, and that means you have to secure it to the skin unless the client plans to sit around and not move during that time. Movement can damage the image, so sealing it will help to prevent that from happening. There's a pretty wide variety of sealing options, so you may want to play with a few of them before deciding what works best for you.

LEMON SUGAR

A mixture of lemon juice and sugar is an inexpensive and effective sealant, but it has its share of complications. If it's too wet, it can turn your dried henna to mush. Plus, in certain climates, the sugar can attract flying insects. But I used this method successfully for a couple of years before I learned about other means. If you want to give it a try, put some sugar in a small saucepan and add just enough lemon juice to make it wet. Then cook it on low to medium heat until it is a thick, syrupy substance. Allow it to cool, and then you can use the end of a cotton swab to carefully dab it onto the henna. Don't actually touch the cotton swab to the henna; let the syrup touch the henna and disperse on its own.

HAIRSPRAY

The simplest thing you can use that most of us have on hand already is hairspray. It supplies a light, fine, sticky mist that seals in the henna

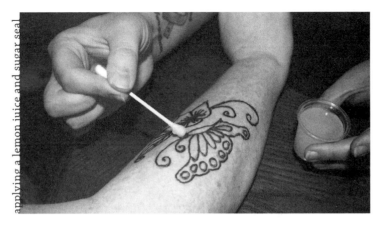

applying a lemon juice and sugar seal

quite effectively. I suggest at least two thin applications, allowing it to dry thoroughly in between.

LIQUID BANDAGE

Spray-on liquid bandaging is also a great option for sealing your henna design. I also recommend two applications of this product, allowing it to dry thoroughly after each layer.

PEEL-OFF FACIAL MASK GEL

I like this option because when you peel it off, the henna comes off with it—no fuss, no muss. But it can pull hairs if you didn't shave them ahead of time, and too much movement can dislodge the dried gel before the paste is ready to be removed. It should be used only in an area where there isn't too much body movement.

LIQUID LATEX

It's an option, but I personally don't recommend it because latex allergies are prevalent and there are plenty of other choices available.

PAPER MEDICAL TAPE

Not the most comfortable option, but very effective and safe for those with sensitive skin. Medical tape will hold the design in place and even allow you to put socks on over foot designs. This method is also recommended for children and pregnant women.

> *TIP:* In addition to a plain sealant, glitter and stick-on decals can be used on or around the henna design to add a little flair. The paste design can be just as beautiful as the stain it produces, and since it has to be worn for several hours, it might as well look great unless you plan to wrap it up.

After your sealant is dry, you can send your recipient on their merry way and instruct them on how to care for their new henna, or you can wrap them up. Wrapping helps to insulate the skin and uses body heat to further enhance the stain potential. Obviously, not all body parts can be wrapped—this is primarily for hand and foot designs. Tissue is placed between the fingers or toes, and then the hand or foot is wrapped with gauze, tissue, or linen. Then that is wrapped with Saran wrap to hold in body heat. Since the hands and feet generally stain so well, this is a very involved process to go through and I don't recommend it unless the client has a history of not being able to achieve a good stain. Also, if too much heat is generated and the person sweats, it could ruin the design.

৬ Henna Aftercare

Caring for henna is actually very simple; it's not like tattoo or piercing aftercare, where there's a wound to heal. So the rules are pretty basic.

- Try not to ruin the pattern. Excessive movement or bumping into things could create cracks in the henna, smoosh it, and move it into areas where it isn't supposed to be, or even rub some of it off. The sealant will help protect it to an extent, but you still have to be careful.
- Don't be impatient. Leave the paste on for at least four hours, but twelve

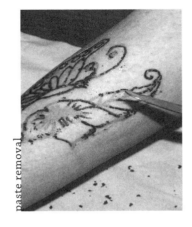
paste removal

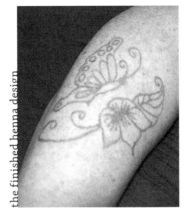
the finished henna design

would be even better. If you want a good stain, you need to be willing to wait and let the lawsone do its job.

- When it's time to remove the paste, do not use any liquids or try to rub it off. Use the back side of a butter knife and gently scrape off as much as you can, unless it was sealed with facial mask gel, in which case it will probably just peel off. If scraping doesn't remove all of the paste, use some olive oil. Rub the oil around to loosen the paste and then gently wipe it off with a soft cloth or paper towel.

- Avoid using soap and water on the stain as long as you can. Eventually, though, you're going to have to wash, so just be careful and don't scrub. The more you wash over the next week or so, the quicker the stain will fade. Put a thin layer of olive or vegetable oil over the design before showering or bathing.

- Shaving, exfoliating, and using petroleum products will all contribute to the fading of your henna design. Avoid them as much as you can.

- All of the things I said to avoid can actually help remove the stain if you decide you don't want it anymore.

If you miss your henna once it's gone, you can just grab some more paste and do it again! The evanescence of the henna stain is part of its beauty, which you can enjoy over and over again.

body painting and special effects

Usually, the only time we think about applying paint to our bodies is for Halloween or to show support for our favorite sports team. But body paint can be a lot of fun any time of the year, whether you have artistic ability or not. It's a great creative outlet, and it's completely safe as long as you use face and/or body paints that are FDA approved and hypoallergenic. After that, you're limited only by your own imagination. You can try out some tattoo ideas you've been thinking about or just go crazy and cover your whole body in color. And all you have to do to erase the whole thing is take a shower. No pain, no permanence, and no commitment—just fun!

What if you were given the opportunity to paint someone else's body? Could you envision something that isn't yet there, as if they are simply a blank canvas waiting to be turned into a masterpiece? There are some extremely talented artists out there who do just that, and one of them is my friend Lisa Berczel.

Lisa and her husband, Lee, own Battledress Paint -n- Body in Corona, California. Lisa had been a graphic artist for over two decades when she began doing airbrush painting as a hobby, in 2003. After a year of painting motorcycles and other nonbreathing surfaces, she decided to give body painting a try when a friend of hers, photographer Adam Chilson, asked her to paint some of his models for a photo shoot. Realizing she had a knack for this unique style of art, she has devoted much of her time to perfecting it. Only a few years into her tenure as a body painter, she has already gone above and beyond what is expected even of more-experienced artists.

I had the pleasure of spending a day with Lisa, watching her prepare her model, Frenzy, for a photo shoot with Chad Michael Ward. While she worked, she filled me in on many of the details that surround this business, both good and bad.

ᴄᴐ Safety First

Body painting may not be nearly as dangerous as puncturing someone's skin or applying a permanent tattoo, but that doesn't mean it's without its share of risks. Lisa's top priority above all else is safety. When she meets a new model, she'll spend a good fifteen minutes talking with them and going over possible allergies, medical history, like asthma and bronchitis (since there is a considerable amount of vapors and not a lot of airflow in the paint booth), and even food allergies.

She'll also make sure that they have eaten, since eating disorders tend to be common among models. A typical paint session can last five to eight hours, which is then followed by a photo shoot, film scene, or live event. After models spend hours around paint vapors and standing for much of the painting process, it's not unheard of for them to faint if they haven't eaten. Lisa says, "Having a model collapse during a live demonstration after you just got through explaining how important it is to make sure your models eat doesn't make a very good impression!"

The last important detail when it comes to safety is the products used on the person serving as the canvas, whom we'll simply refer to as the "model." Although professional modeling experience is not necessarily required, it does help because being painted for hours on end and then performing or posing for lengthy productions and/or photo shoots can take a physical and mental toll. Paints, glues, prosthetics, and anything else that comes in direct contact with the model's lungs or skin must be safe. While some body painters may claim that the paints they use are safe because they are labeled "nontoxic," Lisa only uses paints that are approved for cosmetic use, which have a much shorter list of potential allergens. Many paints contain flexors or binders that give them the ability to stick to fabric, plastics, or other nonliving surfaces. Lisa told the story of a man she knew who had his back painted with fabric paint. Six months later, the pattern from the paint was still visible because of the chemical burns it left behind. Another body painter used rubber cement to glue gems on a model's body. It trapped all the gas vapors from the cement drying between the jewel and the skin and left third-degree chemical burns. And even though Lisa is the first to admit that these instances are rare, she says that when something does go wrong, it's usually really bad.

> *TIP*: *Don't be fooled just because a product claims to be nontoxic. Basically, all that means is that it isn't poison, so it won't kill you if you eat it. But that doesn't mean it's safe or that there won't be any adverse side effects from coming into contact with it. Many of Lisa's earlier models had allergic reactions to the tattoo markers made for children, silicone, and latex. There's also a difference between having something on your skin for a few minutes and having it there for several hours, which painted models have to endure.*

⁓ Skill Requirements

You don't have to have a degree or special certifications to be a body painter, but as much experience and training in art as possible are always best. It's a competitive business, and as most artistic careers go, it's a feast-or-famine kind of job.

Exploring many different fields of art can help you build on a career in body painting. Even though she started using only an airbrush, now Lisa incorporates many different styles into her work and is always challenging herself to try something new. She says, "There's so much to learn from each and every discipline. I've got water-painting books just because of how they use the salt sprinkles and things like that to build texture. I'll see something that I like—say, Chinese brush painting—and think, *How do I get that effect?* I can usually figure out a way to adapt it to what I do."

It's also important to become intimately acquainted with the products that you use for different effects and styles, which can take years of experimenting, and trying many different brands to discover what works best. Since Lisa started her venture into body painting, she has tried many different products. She found that no one particular brand makes everything exactly right for her needs, so her supplies consist of a wide range of products that each serve a different purpose. This experimental phase will also help you build experience as you play around with different products. If you just need a place to start experimenting, though, one of Lisa's favorite companies is Wolfe Face Art & FX. She uses its water-based makeup to apply details by hand.

Just painting alone isn't the only skill needed in this business. Since most models are being painted for television, film, or photographs, the special lighting they're going to be exposed to can enhance or ruin all of your hard work. An understanding of photography and lighting is also essential so that you can anticipate how the things you paint will look once your model is in their assigned venue. Doing test shots throughout the process helps tremendously and can save hours of rework or photo editing.

৯৩ The Model

It's kind of hard to do body painting without a body to paint on, so Lisa recruits models from all over the L.A. area to "wear" her painted costumes. For this session, she called on a young man she has worked with before who goes by the stage name Frenzy.

Frenzy is in his mid-twenties and lives in the L.A. area, where he has been getting steadily more work as his exposure increases. He has a four-year bachelor of arts degree in acting from Cal Poly Pomona and has done a variety of performance arts, such as local theater, runway modeling, and a few minor roles on television drama series, such as Showtime's *Californication* and CW's *90210*.

Frenzy turned out to be the perfect model/actor for this project. He was very patient and followed all the direction that was given to him by Lisa during the six-hour-long painting session. Since they had worked together before, the atmosphere was one of friendship, rather than just painter and model, but both of them took the work they were there to do very seriously. Frenzy chatted blithely with us as he stood outside wearing nothing but a thong as layers upon layers of cold paint coated his skin. And yet, in less than a moment, this genial young man could throw himself into his role and assume a pose with a menacing glint in his eyes that still haunts me to this day. That, my friends, is art.

✺ Body Mapping

Before Lisa actually starts officially painting her planned design on the model, she does something she calls body mapping. Not all painters do this, but that's one of the things that helps her make her designs as technically excellent as possible. Being a former graphic designer, she has an eye for this kind of thing, and that's what makes her stand out despite her relative newness.

Body mapping consists of making simple lines on the model and creating a "blueprint" for the final design. During this stage, Lisa considers every fold, every line, and every seam that will be exposed during the model's assignment. During the day I spent with her, she must have spent an hour just contemplating the final design by painting a few foundation lines on Frenzy and then having him assume a variety of poses so she could see how his muscles and skin would react to the movement. Since the project on this day was to create a straitjacket on Frenzy, it was

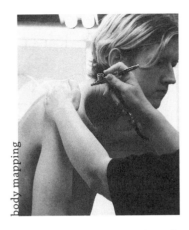

body mapping

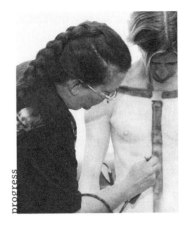

progress

important to plan how to place the straps and how the stitched seams would lay across his shoulders if they were real. Earlier that week, Lisa had already done extensive research on straitjackets and how they work.

Not all body painting involves creating a clothing facade, although Lisa does a lot of wardrobe design in her line of work. Sometimes the event simply requires a theme or a feel and leaves her open to a wider creative avenue. In this case, she says, it can actually be more challenging because she has to create something that doesn't actually exist.

∽ Getting Down to Business

Once she's ready to get down to start the actual painting, Lisa has to decide whether to use water- or alcohol-based paint, or a combination of both. Alcohol-based paint is rewettable, and it bleeds and seeps into other colors like watercolor paints do. Water-based airbrush paint has a matte, flat finish, and appears softer to the camera.

Once Lisa got an opaque white foundation on Frenzy's frame, it was time to start creating the details of the straitjacket. The straps and any shadows were done with the airbrush, while individual creases, stitching in the straps, and the metal rings were done by hand with brushes. Every time I thought she couldn't possibly make it look any better than it already did, she'd add a tiny detail that would make it stand out even more.

She also incorporated a few straps made of paper that she painted to match the ones she painted on Frenzy. The paper straps were glued to Frenzy's skin in a few places and allowed to hang, or were used to wrap around his hands, completing the three-dimensional look of the one-dimensional painted straitjacket.

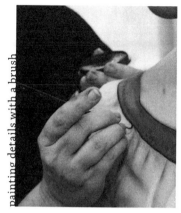
painting details with a brush

ᥱᕋ Dealing with Obstacles

When you're working on a human canvas, there are obstacles you have to learn to overcome that traditional painters don't have to worry about. If the model sweats, which is kind of hard to avoid, the paint can smudge. If they fall down or something gets spilled on them, an entire section of the paint can be ruined. If they get sick, the "canvas" may not be able to attend its own showing.

Lisa says she loves absolutely everything about her job, but that doesn't mean it doesn't have its share of ups and downs. You just simply have to be able to roll with the punches.

It also helps to have a "right hand" that can help out, especially in an emergency situation. Lisa's husband, Lee, is the other half of Battledress and the one who handles the unglamorous but vital details. Lee gets handed bottles to shake and airbrushes to unclog. He also has to improvise on the spot, creating technical solutions for unpredictable situations. (*"Can you make fake nipple rings?" "Why, yes. YES, we can."*) Lisa is usually the one who gets the media attention because she's the one behind the airbrush, but she readily admits she'd be lost without her go-to man!

ᥱᕋ Special Effects Makeup by Michael Mosher

After the painting was finished, the next step for Frenzy was to have his hair and makeup done to reflect the crazy asylum patient he was being transformed into. That was a job for Hollywood's own Michael Mosher,

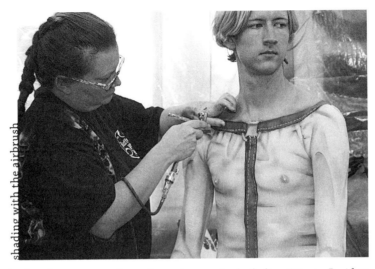

shading with the airbrush

who has done stage makeup for major movies including *Titanic*, *Resident Evil 3*, and *Pirates of the Caribbean: At World's End*.

Michael has been doing makeup for a living since 1991, but he says it's really the only thing he's wanted to do since he was seven years old. He lived on *Fangoria* magazine, watched *Creature Double Feature* religiously, and dreamed of creating monsters from a young age.

He started out doing makeup at an opera house in San Diego. After doing that for a while, he moved to Los Angeles and managed to hook up with a great production company that gave him his big break. Now, as Frenzy said, "Michael is one of the best, if not *the* best, in Hollywood."

The only thing Michael regrets is not going to cosmetology school, because he really enjoys doing hair as well as makeup. If this is the kind of business you want to break into, cosmetology schooling is highly recommended. Not everyone falls into a great position like Michael did, and the more you have to offer, the better your odds of being noticed are.

The project had two objectives: One set of photos would be done from the viewers' perspective, while the other would be done from Frenzy's. So, in addition to adding some bruiselike coloring to Frenzy's face and teasing his hair out to look like it hadn't been combed or washed in months, Michael glued

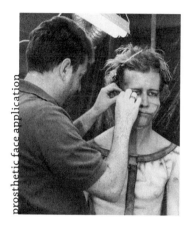

prosthetic face application

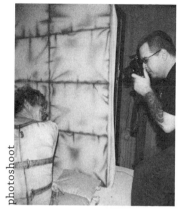

photoshoot

on a wide prosthetic mouth that took Frenzy to a whole new level of dementia. Add in Frenzy's great acting skills, and the asylum patient was complete.

✎ The Photo Shoot—Enter Chad Michael Ward

All the work that went into creating the perfect model would have been kind of pointless without a great setting to place him in. Lisa, Lee, and Frenzy all worked on a large, forced-perspective box that had pillowlike squares painted inside to look like padded walls. A padded mattress cover was placed on the floor of the box, and when Frenzy climbed inside and sat down, he looked like a demented clown in a padded cell—exactly the effect everyone was going for.

Now it was time for the whole day's work to come to fruition. They had the model, they had the set—all they needed was someone to take the pictures. Enter Chad Michael Ward, L.A.'s finest fantasy and horror photographer.

Chad has a very unique style of photography because he combines his photos with digital artistry to create stunning—not to mention chilling—visual effects. He's been working as a professional photographer for over thirteen years, but has also delved into other artistic venues during that time. He especially enjoys directing and has directed music videos for Slash, Billy Idol, and Marilyn Manson. While doing pro-

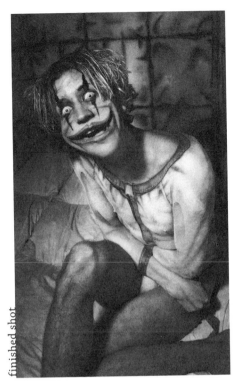
finished shot

duction design and promo posters for *The Gene Generation,* Chad hooked up with producer Pearry Reginald Teo and they formed Teo/Ward Productions. In everything that he does, Chad sticks with what he loves most: the dark and macabre.

When Lisa proposed the asylum theme to Chad and asked if he'd be interested, he was intrigued. Once he got to the set, he was in his element. He spent hours on the set, experimenting with different effects, including some black-light scenes with glow paint. If Frenzy didn't look creepy enough to begin with, once Chad was done adding his digital voodoo, he definitely looked like something straight out of a horror film.

So, as you can see, body art isn't all just about tattoos and piercings. From beginning to end, this entire production was full of many different styles of body art: modeling, acting, body painting, special effects make-up, hair design, and photography. Anything that decorates, enhances, or transforms the human body can be considered body art. Whether you're the artist or the canvas, it's all about finding a way to express yourself.

state laws

The following list will give you the last known age requirement laws for tattoo and body piercings in each of the United States. Please be aware that these laws are ever changing, so if you need to know the age requirements for a particular city or state, it's best to call one of the studios in the area and check with them to be sure of the most current laws. Also, many states allows city and county governments to create their own mandates that may override the state laws. This list should be used as a reference only.

State	Tattoo Age of Consent	Tattoo Age Minimum w/ Parental Consent	Piercing Age of Consent	Piercing Age Minimum w/ Parental Consent
Alabama	18	None	18	None
Alaska	18	No Provision	18	None
Arizona	18	14	18	14
Arkansas	18	16	18	16
California	18	No Provision	18	None
Colorado	18	16	18	16
Connecticut	18	16	18	None

State	Tattoo Age of Consent	Tattoo Age Minimum w/ Parental Consent	Piercing Age of Consent	Piercing Age Minimum w/ Parental Consent
Delaware	18	None	18	None
Florida	18	16	18	None
Georgia	18	No Provision	18	14
Hawaii	18	None	None	None
Idaho	18	14	18	14
Illinois	18	No Provision	18	No Provision
Indiana	18	None	18	None
Iowa	18	No Provision	18	No Provision (Except Earlobes)
Kansas	18	None	18	None
Kentucky	18	None	18	None
Louisiana	18	None	18	None
Maine	18	No Provision	18	No Provision
Maryland	18	None	18	None
Mass.	18	No Provision	18	None
Michigan	18	None	18	None
Minnesota	18	None	18	None
Mississippi	18	No Provision	18	No Provision
Missouri	18	None	18	None
Montana	18	None	18	None
Nebraska	18	None	18	None
Nevada	18	None	18	None
New Hampshire	18	No Provision	18	None
New Jersey	18	None	18	None

State	Tattoo Age of Consent	Tattoo Age Minimum w/ Parental Consent	Piercing Age of Consent	Piercing Age Minimum w/ Parental Consent
New Mexico	18	None	18	None
New York	18	No Provision	18	No Provision
North Carolina	18	No Provision	18	14
North Dakota	18	None	18	None
Ohio	18	None	18	None
Oklahoma	18	No Provision	18	None
Oregon	18	No Provision	18	No Provision
Pennsylvania	18	None	18	None
Rhode Island	18	No Provision	18	None
South Carolina	21	18	18	No Provision
South Dakota	18	None	18	None
Tennessee	18	16	18	16
Texas	18	None	18	None
Utah	18	None	18	None
Vermont	18	None	18	None
Virginia	18	None	18	None
Washington	18	No Provision	18	None
West Virginia	18	None	18	None
Wisconsin	18	No Provision	18	16
Wyoming	18	None	18	None

lexicon

Autoclave: A sterilizing machine that is designed to kill harmful bacteria on the surfaces of reusable tools, such as piercing needles and tattoo machine tubes. Autoclaves must be tested regularly to ensure that they are killing all pathogenic spores effectively.

Anodization: The process of exposing something to an electrical charge after dipping it into an acidic solution. Niobium and titanium body jewelry are often anodized to produce a variety of different-colored jewelry.

Biomechanical: A type of art that depicts creatures or images that have both biological and mechanical components. H. R. Giger is a well-known biomechanical artist.

Blowout: A term used to describe the halo effect that occurs around a tattoo because the ink was deposited too deeply or at too much of an angle, so that the ink settled in a different location from that of the original line.

Carrier solution: A variety of liquids that can be mixed with pigments to create a more workable product that inhibits the growth of bacteria and prevents the powdered pigment from clumping up. Some examples are distilled water, witch hazel, and glycerin.

CDC: An acronym for the Centers for Disease Control and Prevention. The CDC is a division of the U.S. federal government that has much influence on the practices of regulated tattoo and piercing establishments.

Collector: Someone who gets a significant number of tattoos and enjoys "collecting" these many pieces of art.

Cover-up: A tattoo that is applied over an already existing tattoo in order to cover or camouflage it.

Crusties: Dried lymph and sebum that surround a new piercing and feel a bit like grains of sand. This is perfectly normal for a couple of weeks after getting a piercing.

Custom: A tattoo design that is created specifically for the client, rather than something that is copied from a preexisting tattoo pattern.

Dermis: The innermost layer of skin that contains the connective tissue between the epidermis and the hypodermis. The dermis contains hair follicles, sweat and sebaceous glands, lymph and blood vessels, and nerve endings. It is within this dermal layer that tattoo ink settles and holds firm.

Disposable: Tools used for creating tattoos or piercings that are not reusable because they can't be sterilized. Disposable items that come into contact with bodily fluids are considered hazardous waste and must be treated as such.

Endorphins: Hormonal peptides that, in response to pain or stress (both good and bad), attach themselves to opiate receptors in the brain. This reduces pain by creating a euphoric response, nicknamed "runner's high," to describe the sensation experienced by runners who push themselves beyond their normal threshold.

Epidermis: The outermost layer of skin that is constantly regenerating and protects our bodies from outside elements.

Fistula: The tunnel or passage that exists between two opening points, such as with a piercing that passes through the skin.

Flash: Drawings of tattoo-ready designs that are typically seen hanging up in tattoo shops for perusal by patrons.

Frenulum: A thin piece of connective tissue that restricts movement of an organ or muscle, such as the frenulum under your tongue that connects it to the floor of your mouth.

Gauge: A unit of measurement used to describe the thickness of body piercing needles and the corresponding jewelry.

Hyperpigmentation: An overabundance of pigment in the skin that results in a darker appearance than that of the surrounding areas. Sometimes called "sun spots" because they're often caused by sun damage.

Hypodermis: The subcutaneous fat layer that creates a cushion between the skin and muscles. A hypodermic needle seeks to reach this region to deliver medication, because it is then carried to the rest of the body. If tattoo ink were deposited this deeply, it would also travel, creating a blowout, or be carried away completely.

Hypopigmentation: The loss of pigment in the skin that results in a lighter appearance than that of the surrounding areas. This is usually due to some kind of tissue damage and/or scarring.

Keloid: A buildup of excess scar tissue due to a condition that causes the body to overproduce corrective tissue when it has been damaged. While an undesirable response to a body piercing or tattoo, minor keloiding is the goal of intentional scarification.

Lymph: A clearish liquid that's sometimes released from the body as a result of a puncture wound, such as a piercing. When dry, it forms "crusties" that build up around the piercing site.

Micropigmentation: A technical term for permanent cosmetics and areola reconstruction through the process of tattooing pigment underneath the skin.

Modified: The term some people prefer to use for themselves when they alter their body in one way or another, particularly through more extreme methods than just tattoos or piercings.

MRSA: An acronym for "methicillin resistant staphylococcus aureus," MRSA (pronounced "MER-suh") is a very resilient strain of staph bacteria that isn't easily killed with the usual round of antibiotics.

Neo-tribalism: An abstract type of tattoo style that imitates primitive works of swirls, curved lines, and geometric shapes but doesn't have any cultural significance.

New school: The latest trends in tattoo design that share such characteristics as bold lines, bright secondary and tertiary colors, and whatever technique may be popular at the time.

Old school: Also simply called "traditional" style, old-school tattoos imitate the style that first became popular in Western culture. The tattoos are characterized by the use of primary colors, thick outlines, and simple drawings with dramatic highlights.

Oxidization: When something has a chemical reaction to oxygen exposure. Rust is an example of oxidization.

Pathogen: A harmful microorganism that causes disease, such as bacteria or a virus.

Perichondritis: An infection of the connective tissue that surrounds the cartilage of the ear. It's the most common infection from cartilage piercings and can cause severe damage to the cartilage itself.

Pigment: A powder made from various materials, such as iron oxide, to create a base for permanent-cosmetics colors and tattoo "ink." The powder is then suspended in a carrier solution to create a thin paste or liquid.

Regulated: When a city, state, or province has laws that control how tattoo and piercing establishments must be run and conducts inspections to ensure those laws are being followed.

Scar: Corrective tissue that is formed by new cells when the original tissue was damaged.

Sebum: An oily substance that can build up around a piercing site along with lymph. When exposed to bacteria it can give off a bad odor.

Scratcher: A person who tattoos under unsterile conditions and has no concern for the law or client safety.

Standard Precautions: Formerly called Universal Precautions, they are the sterile procedures the CDC requires anyone working in a biohazardous environment to follow.

Suspension: A performance art and spiritual experience in which a participant is hung from large hooks pierced through their body.

Tebori: An ancient form of Japanese hand tattooing that uses a group of needles tied to the end of a stick or rod. A handful of artists still practice this art form today, but with some modern improvements in sterilization practices.

Touch-up: Having a new tattoo cleaned up to fill in any lines or color missing after the first session, or having an old tattoo recolored to return it to its original luster and sharpness.

Tribal: A tattoo that is an authentic cultural tattoo from a tribal community, such as the signature Samoan *pe'a* (full-body tattoo) or Maori *moko* (facial tattoo). What many people refer to as "tribal" is actually *neo-tribal* art.

resources

ALLIANCE OF PROFESSIONAL TATTOOISTS

Formed in 1992, this nonprofit organization was created to raise the bar of tattoo safety practices in the industry. Now, APT membership is somewhat of an honor badge worn by tattoo artists who follow the safety standards they have established. (www.safe-tattoos.com)

ASSOCIATION OF PROFESSIONAL PIERCERS

The APP is considered the highest authority on body piercing procedure and safety. The nonprofit organization was formed in 1994 to bring safety awareness to the industry and its advocates. (www.safepiercing.org)

BODIES OF SUBVERSION: A SECRET HISTORY OF WOMEN AND TATTOO (2ND EDITION)

This is an amazing history book that introduces you to the women who helped to establish a female presence in a male-dominated industry. From the heavily tattooed sideshow beauties of the early twentieth century to today's most influential female tattoo artists, author Margot Mifflin covers them all. (powerHouse Books, second edition—April 9, 2001—ISBN-10: 189045110X)

BORIS VALLEJO

Tattoo renditions of the dynamic fantasy art of Boris Vallejo have been highly sought after by fans of both art forms. It's hard not to find yourself catching your breath as you tour the countless pages of Vallejo's paintings on his website. (www.imaginistix.com)

COOPSTUFF

Although he's primarily referred to as a hot-rod artist, the renderings of Christopher "Coop" Cooper have long been favored by tattoo fans, particularly his sexy devil-girl creations. If you want something naughty in nature, you might be interested in taking a look at Coop's online store, which features a pretty good collection of his art. (www.coopstuff.com)

CSYMBOL (CHINESE CHARACTERS)

If you need an accurate and trustworthy translation of a word or phrase into the Chinese language, Jun Shan is your man. He's actually a former colleague of mine, and I trust Jun implicitly for his Chinese translations. He also has some cool personalized products that feature popular Chinese phrases, and all of his prices are very reasonable. (www.csymbol.com)

HANZI SMATTER

This is a humorous but useful website that exposes some of the embarrassing mistranslations of Asian languages, particularly in tattoos. Most people who write in to the blog's owner, Tian, find out that their tattoo doesn't mean what it was supposed to. Learning from others' mistakes is a lot less expensive and embarrassing than finding out your kanji "friendship" tattoo actually says "sesame chicken." (www.hanzismatter.com)

HELL CITY TATTOO CONVENTION

Absolutely my favorite tattoo show, now in both "Killumbus," Ohio, and Phoenix, Arizona. (www.hellcity.com)

HOW TATTOOS WORK

As part of the HowStuffWorks entity, this article gives a great synopsis of how tattoos are applied, including an animated display of the ink being deposited underneath the skin. It also explains the workings of the tattoo machine itself and why it's able to move the needle so quickly. (www.howstuffworks.com/tattoo.htm)

INTERNATIONAL TATTOO ART MAGAZINE

This is a very well-balanced magazine that features informative articles and beautiful photos of tattoos done by artists from all over the world. This magazine gives you a broader exposure to the world of tattoos than any other publication does. (www.internationaltattooart.com)

LUIS ROYO

The fantasy works of the Spanish artist Luis Royo are among my personal favorites. Royo incorporates tattoos, piercings, and other forms of body art into his beautiful subjects, but he does it with a futuristic edge. (www.luisroyo.com)

MARK RYDEN

I wouldn't care to venture into the mind of this artist, but I can't deny that his disturbing-yet-intriguing renderings of childlike creatures make for some of the most interesting and colorful tattoos I've ever seen. (www.markryden.com)

NATIONAL TATTOO ASSOCIATION

The NTA is dedicated to raising the bar in regard to the quality of tattoo artistry. It hosts a fantastic convention, in a different location every year, that features only the best artists in the world. Membership is limited, but anyone can attend the convention as a visitor. (www. nationaltattooassociation.com)

NATIONAL GEOGRAPHIC

Both the magazine and the online version have featured numerous articles about tattoo culture and history in all parts of the world. This is a great resource for unbiased information about the beginnings of tattoo and body piercing practices. (www.nationalgeographic.com)

NATURAL EXPRESSIONS

My favorite henna/mehndi supply company. High-quality henna powders, pre-mixed pastes, and applicators. (www.naturalexpression.com)

RED CROSS UNIVERSAL PRECAUTIONS COURSE

This is an online course that is provided to both professionals and enthusiasts of the body art industry. It's good to know what practices are expected of your artist, and the things you'll learn in this course can help in anti-everyday-cross-contamination efforts as well. You will receive a certificate upon passing the online test. (www .redcrossonlinetraining.org)

SKIN & INK MAGAZINE

Skin & Ink is one of my favorite tattoo magazines. It focuses less on tattoo photos (although you do get a nice display of those, too) and more on the culture and the people who have been influential in tattoo history. It's a great, "meaty" magazine with no fillers. (www.skinink.com)

TATTOO ARCHIVE

This is my favorite source for tattoo history, especially if you're looking for information about a specific person. Through this website, you can also join the Paul Rogers Tattoo Research Center, a nonprofit organization that was designed to help preserve tattoo history. (www.tattooarchive.com)

TATTOO HISTORY: A SOURCE BOOK

This book, although a little bit disorganized in its arrangement, is probably the ultimate authority on tattoo history. The author, Steve Gilbert, was able to compile an immense collection of documents, drawings, and photos that span thousands of years. (powerHouse Books—February, 2001)

TATTOODLES

With a paid monthly or yearly subscription, you have access to hundreds of high-quality tattoo designs if you're in need of inspiration. Unlike random flash sheets, the drawings are divided into easily searchable categories so you can narrow down your search much more quickly. (www .tattoodles.com)

THE VANISHING TATTOO

This online museum is full of articles and pictures, and has an absorbing virtual tour of the evolution of tattoo art from ancient to modern times. While searching for the few remaining authentic tattoos in today's world, Thomas Lockhart takes you on his amazing journeys across the globe. (www.vanishingtattoo.com)

WORLD OF FROUD

Brian Froud is one of the top fairy artists in the world, and his creatures are very popular as tattoos. In addition to the Froud family website, I highly recommend Brian's book, *Brian Froud's World of Faerie,* which you can get a sneak peek of on the site. (www.worldoffroud.com)

sources by chapter

CHAPTER 1. WHAT IS A TATTOO?

- www.tattooarchive.com
- www.designboom.com/history/tattoo_history.html
- www.vanishingtattoo.com/tattoo_museum/history.html
- www.powerverbs.com/tattooyou/history.htm
- www.pbs.org/skinstories/history/index.html
- Gilbert, Steve. *Tattoo History: A Source Book* (New York: powerHouse Books, 2001).
- Krakow, Amy. *The Total Tattoo Book* (New York: Grand Central Publishing, 1994).
- Mifflin, Margo. *Bodies of Subversion: A Secret History of Women and Tattoo* (New York: powerHouse Books, 2001).
- Miller, Jean-Chris. *The Body Art Book: A Complete, Illustrated Guide to Tattoos, Piercings, and Other Body Modification* (New York: Berkley Trade, 2004).

CHAPTER 2. 120 YEARS OF TATTOO EVOLUTION

- www.tattooarchive.com/history/coleman_august_cap.htm
- www.tattooarchive.com/history/sailor_tattoos.htm
- www.tattooarchive.com/history/tattoo_machine.htm
- Gilbert, Steve. *Tattoo History*
- Krakow, Amy. *The Total Tattoo Book*
- Mifflin, Margo. *Bodies of Subversion*
- Miller, Jean-Chris. *The Body Art Book*

CHAPTER 6. RELIGIOUS, SOCIAL, AND EMPLOYMENT CONFLICTS

- www.hillel.org/about/news/2007/jan/tattooed_22Jan2007
- www.nytimes.com/2008/07/17/fashion/17SKIN.html
- www.cityfile.com/dailyfile/932

CHAPTER 21. LIFETIME MAINTENANCE

- www.dermatology.about.com/cs/skincareproducts/a/spf.htm
- www.pediatrics.about.com/od/sunscreen/a/sunscreen_myths.htm

CHAPTER 28. THE RISKS OF BODY PIERCING

- www.danaid.com
- www.irwinmitchell.com/PressOffice/PressReleases
- www.thestar.co.uk/news/Death-of-teen-sparks-new.1852662.jp
- www.telegraph.co.uk/news/uknews
- http://news.bbc.co.uk/2/hi/uk_news/england
- www.americanheart.org/presenter.jhtml?identifier=1310
- www.mayoclinic.com/health/tricuspid-atresia/DS00796
- http://emedicine.medscape.com/article/158359-overview
- www.americanheart.org/presenter.jhtml?identifier=4436
- www.mayoclinic.com/health/endocarditis/DS00409
- http://www.hse.gov.uk/lau/lacs
- www.thepaper24-7.com

- www.bio-medicine.org/medicine-news/Piercing-breast-led-to-mastecto
  my-in-teenager-15424-1
- www.thepaper24-7.com
- www.nnff.org

CHAPTER 30. TYPES OF BODY JEWELRY
- www.azom.com/details.asp?ArticleID=1558
- www.ezinearticles.com/?Testing-Silver-and-Silver-Grades&id=411984
- www.plastomertech.com/ptfeproperties.htm

CHAPTER 39. PIERCING FAQS
- www.safety-council.org/news/media/releases/2007/Lightning.html

CHAPTER 42.
IMPLANTS AND EXTREME MODIFICATIONS
- http://news.bmezine.com/2007/07/02/three-blind-mice/

CHAPTER 43. MEHNDI—THE ART OF HENNA PAINTING
- www.hennapage.com/henna/history/index.html
- www.mehendiworld.com/mehendi-history.html
- www.ragani.com/henna/history.html
- www.hc-sc.gc.ca/sr-sr/finance
- www.foxnews.com/story/0,2933,346090,00.html
- www.metro.co.uk/news
- www.news.com.au/perthnow
- www.canada.com/ch/cheknews
- www.foxnews.com/story/0,2933,431241,00.html
- www.wbaltv.com/news/13636338
- www.snopes.com/horrors/vanities/henna.asp

photo credits

middle right (Mehndi), artist: Dawn Grace of Tattoo Factory in Chicago, IL.

bottom left (black and gray), photo © Don Hudson. artist: Brian Benner of Truth & Triumph in Dayton, Ohio. model: Mike Harwat.

bottom right (realism), photo © Don Hudson. artist: Justin Wright of Tattoo Alley in Akron, Ohio. model: Elisa Miller.

pages 72-74: photos © Karen Hudson. artist: Amanda Cancilla. model: Stephanie Ellis.

page 89: © Karen Hudson.

page 97: photo © Don Hudson. artist: David Villard of Renaissance Tattoo in Woonsocket, RI. model: Wolfie.

page 99: photo © Don Hudson. model: Don Hudson.

page 102: photos © Thomas Randall. cover-up artist: Thomas Randall.

page 104: photos courtesy of Alma Lasers, www.almalasers.com. removal performed by Prof Arie Orenstein, Tel_Aviv, Israel.

pages 107-109: all photos © Don Hudson. page 107, right: Kim Garcia's tattoos by artist Dave "Byrd" Klaiber.

page 117: photo © Domini Dragoone. Thanks to Body Manipulations, www.bodym.com. model: Paul Stoll.

pages 134-135: photos © Domini Dragoone. Thanks to Body Manipulations, www.bodym.com.

page 137: left, photo © Domini Dragoone, model: Carmen Carrasco. right, photo © Singer Blake, model: Singer Blake.

page 138: photos © Domini Dragoone, models: top left, Apaulo Hart. top right, anonymous.

page 141-143: photos © Domini Dragoone. Thanks to Body Manipulations, www.bodym.com.

page 145: photos © Don Hudson. models: left, Midny Messer. right, Alex Benoit.

page 147: left, photo © Domini Dragoone. right, photo © Singer Blake, model: Singer Blake.

page 148: top and bottom, photos © Singer Blake, model: Singer Blake. middle, photo © Domini Dragoone. Thanks to Body Manipulations, www.bodym.com.

page 151: photos © Domini Dragoone, models: left, Domini Dragoone. right, Steve Joyner.

page 152: photos © Domini Dragoone, models: left, Nick Venn. Piercing done at Body Exotic in San Jose, CA. right, Steve Joyner.

page 155: left, photo © Domini Dragoone. Piercing done at Ancient Art Tattoo in Raonoke Virginia. model : Candice Miller. right, photo © Don Hudson. piercer: Mike Moore of Voodoo Tattoo. model: Justin Rodriguez.

page 156: left, photo © Don Hudson. Piercings done at Artistic Soul in Marion, OH. model: Hope Dean. right, photo © Domini Dragoone. model: Noelle Glenn.

page 157: photos © Domini Dragoone. models (L-R): MizMargo, Carmen Carrasco.

page 158: left photo © Domini Dragoone. model: MizMargo. right, photo © Don Hudson. piercer: William Fecke of Momma's Tattoo. model: Mindy Messer.

page 161: photos © Domini Dragoone. left, piercing done by Christ Scherer of Stained Skin in Columbus, OH. models: left, Jennifer Leddy. right, anonymous.

page 162: photos © Domini Dragoone. models: left, Carmen Carrasco. right, anonymous.

page 164: photos © Domini Dragoone. models: left, Jennifer Williams. right, Steve Joyner.

page 165: photo © Don Hudson. piercer Jason of Downtown Tattoo in Zanesville, OH. model: Maria Kelinert.

page 167: left, photo © Domini Dragoone. piercer: Paul Stoll of Body Manipulations in San Francisco, CA (right nipple only, to match old angled piercing on left nipple). model: Alexei Jacobson. right, photo: Don Hudson. piercer: Mike Miracle of Body Language in Columbus, OH. model: Robyn Zanow.

page 171: photo © Domini Dragoone. Piercing done at Cold Steel in San Francisco, CA. model: MizMargo.

pages 175, 176, 179, 181, and 183: illustrations © Don Hudson, www. visualimpactart.com.

index

from laser removal, 103; from Listerine, 164; from the Madison, 170–171; piercing, 125, 160, 212; stretch marks, 34–35; tattooing over, 16, 35–36, 238; from tattoo removal, 23

school, tattoo, 113

scratchers: defined, 39, 289; vs. professionals, 39–42; Spaulding/Rogers inspire, 12–13; terminology, 45

scratching tattoos, 90

scrotal ladder, 184

scrotum piercing, 183–184

scrumper (upper-lip frenulum/smiley), 165

sea salt soaks, 203, 205, 207, 218

sebum, 289

secrets, from parents, 100

secrets, tattooing, 12

self-cutting, 240–241

self-expression, 15, 50

sensitivity: during menstruation, 113; to nickel, 118, 143, 213–214; to tattooing pain, 19

septicemia, 126, 166, 215

septum piercing, 157–158, 208

sex, oral, 207, 237

Shan, Jun, 292

sharps, 21

shaving, 72, 271

shower scrubbies, 168–169

sickness, 111

silicone jewelry, 146

silver, 144

single point piercings, 171–172

skin: aging, 94; cleansers, 82; and color choice, 53; conditions, pre-existing, 36–38; elasticity, 34; post-surgery healing, 35–36; post-tattoo healing, 79–90;

prepping, 72; regrowth after gauging up, 211; sensitivity, 19, 68, 81, 118, 143; symptoms of healing complications, 213–214; thickness, 18–19

Skin & Ink, 294

skin scribe, 191

smell: of branding flesh, 249; of fresh henna, 261; funky piercing, 220–221; of untainted henna, 259

smiley (scrumper/upper-lip frenulum), 165

smoking, 164, 207

snacking, 20

snake bite piercing, 161–162

soap, 81–82, 202, 271

sobriety, 131–132

social pressure, 26–27

SofTap, 228, 232

Spaulding, Huck, 12, 13

SPF factors, 92

spirals, 137–138

spore tests, 48

SSS (surgical stainless steel), 141–142

Standard Precautions, 31, 41, 55, 129, 130, 290

staph infections, 29–30, 100, 215, 241

state laws, 282–284

stencils, design, 71–72, 73, 242, 266, 267

sterilization: assessing, 47–49, 55; of body jewelry, 145, 146, 147; of cutting equipment, 241; early 20th century ignorance of, 10; as ignored by scratchers, 12–13, 39; of piercing guns, 115; of piercing needles, 117; in professional piercing shops, 129, 190, 191; in professional tattoo shops, 41–42

acknowledgments

Just a few days after I agreed to write *Living Canvas,* my husband was in a serious motorcycle accident. After he spent a week in the hospital and had surgery to repair his shattered hip, knee, and hand, then went through many months of difficult recovery, I'm happy to say that he's doing better than the doctors expected. But the months leading up to this point and the effort required to care for him and write a book at the same time were challenging, to say the very least. Those who had a direct hand in helping me get through the past several months receive more of a standing ovation than just my thanks.

For appearing out of nowhere at exactly the right time, I applaud my agent, Meredith Hays, of FinePrint Literary Management. She stuck with me even through her maternity leave, taking my emails and caring for a new baby at the same time. She probably has the spit-up on her keyboard to prove it.

For being patient with me (and probably pretending she didn't see those moody email responses) when I just wasn't in the right frame of mind to write, and for wisely insisting that we extend my deadline, I applaud my editor, Brooke Warner.

For being my rock, as always, and supporting me any way he could even when his body was broken and bruised, I applaud my husband and best friend, Don. I love you, babe! I also applaud my daughters, Tessa and Ciera, for giving up their vacation time, being so helpful around the house, and taking care of their daddy when I had to write.

For always being supportive of me in all of my endeavors and for not killing me for getting my face tattooed (even though you don't know about it yet), I applaud my loving mother, Bonnie Poynter. (Well, I guess you know about it now, don't you? Love you, Mommy!)

For helping me with my research by providing their expertise and spending countless hours answering all of my questions, I applaud Jane Adler, Lisa and Lee Berczel, Jesse Villemaire, Chad Michael Ward, and Michael Mosher.

For the many hours spent designing and inking many of my favorite tattoos, I applaud Kym Tongate. You rock, lady!

For sharing the stories of their sons and reliving some of the worst days of their lives just so others won't have to go through the same thing, I applaud Jill Hanlin and Christina Anderson.

For their help, support, understanding, and laughter, and for just being the amazing people they are, I applaud Kara and John Pringle, Karri and Bryan Harbert, Karen and Michael Perry, Lacey White, Tammy Shaw, Cristen Potmesil; all of my friends at the Parents of Type 1 Diabetes Support Group (www.type1parents.org); and my True Blue Nation friends: Donna, Rob, Kat, and John. Much love, and go Colts!

Last but not least, for keeping me spiritually grounded and positive during the most stressful moments and for reminding me to breathe, I applaud my dear friend Ms. Mick Michieli-Beasley.

about the author

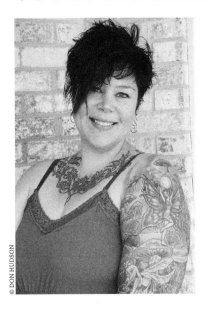

© DON HUDSON

Karen L. Hudson is the coauthor of *Chick Ink: 40 Stories of Tattoos—and the Women Who Wear Them.* She became fascinated with the world of body art at age twenty-three. In 1997, she began an apprenticeship in which she learned not only about the art of tattooing, but also about sterilization and safety issues. Hudson quickly realized that too many people are uninformed before they make the decision to permanently mark or alter their bodies, which influences much of her writing and advocacy today.

As the publisher of the popular website Tattoo.about.com, Hudson serves the community with passion and understanding, always remembering what it was like to be completely new to the world of wearable art. She has been one the world's top body art safety and acceptance advocates since 1999. She lives with her husband and children in Indianapolis, Indiana.

Selected Titles from Seal Press

For more than thirty years, Seal Press has published groundbreaking books. By women. For women. Visit our website at www.sealpress.com. Check out the Seal Press blog at www.sealpress.com/blog

It's So You: 35 Women Write About Personal Expression Through Fashion and Style, edited by Michelle Tea. $15.95, 1-58005-215-0. From the haute couture houses of the ruling class to DIY girls who make restorative clothing and create their own hodgepodge style, this is the first book to explore women's ambivalence toward, suspicion of, indulgence in, and love of fashion on every level.

Offbeat Bride: Taffeta-Free Alternatives for Independent Brides, by Ariel Meadow Stallings. $15.95, 1-58005-180-4. Part memoir and part anecdotal how-to, *Offbeat Bride* is filled with sanity-saving tips, advice, and stories to guide even the most out-there bride.

Rock Your Stars: Your Astrological Guide to Getting It All, by Holiday Mathis. $15.95, 1-58005-217-7. In the lively and intelligent *Rock Your Stars,* syndicated columnist and "rock 'n' roll astrologer" Holiday Mathis offers a modern manual to making every life decision, whether it's what to wear, who to love, which career ladder to climb, what color to paint the bedroom, or how to find the right exercise plan—all by using astrology as a practical guide.

Cinderella's Big Score: Women of the Punk and Indie Underground, by Maria Raha. $17.95, 1-58005-116-2. A tribute to the transgressive women of the underground music scene, who not only rocked as hard as the boys, but also tested the limits of what is culturally acceptable—even in the anarchic world of punk.

The List: 100 Ways to Shake Up Your Life, by Gail Belsky. $15.95, 1-58005-256-8. Get a tattoo, ride in a fire truck, or use food as foreplay— this collection of 100 ideas will inspire women to shake things up and do something they never dared to consider.

About Face: Women Write about What They See When They Look in the Mirror, edited by Anne Burt and Christina Baker Kline. $15.95, 1-58005-246-0. 25 women writers candidly examine their own faces—and each face has a story to tell.